WOM
CANC

WOMEN'S CANCERS

The Treatment Options:
everything you need
to know

DONNA DAWSON

PIATKUS

I dedicate this book with all my love to my mother, Patricia Kirby, who faced ovarian cancer with courage, humour and dignity and, when the odds were down, showed me how to die; and to my stepmother, Gwen Poitras, who fought and won her battle against breast cancer and who shows me how to take life a day at a time . . .

© 1990 Donna Dawson

First published in 1990 by
Judy Piatkus (Publishers) Limited
of 5 Windmill Street, London W1P 1HF

British Library Cataloguing in Publication Data
Dawson, Donna
    Women's cancers.
    I. Women. Cancer
    I. Title
    616.99′4′0088042

    ISBN 0 – 86188 – 955 – X
            0 – 86188 – 966 – 5 (Pbk)

Edited by Ruth Baldwin
Designed by Sue Ryall

Photoset in 11/12 Compugraphic Baskerville by
Action Typesetting Ltd, Gloucester.
Printed and bound in Great Britian by
Billing & Sons Ltd, Worcester

Contents

Contents

ACKNOWLEDGEMENTS

I wish to thank all of the following people and organisations for giving so generously of their time and help in connection with this book:

Dr Ian Jacobs; Dr Tim Oliver, reader in medical oncology; David Oram, gynaecological surgeon; John Shepherd, consultant gynaecological surgeon and oncologist; Professor Martin Vessey; Peter Trott, consultant cytopathologist; Dr Eve Wiltshaw; Professor Michael Baum; Dr Karol Sikora; Dr Lionel Crawford; Dr Ian Fentiman; Dr Peter Mason; Dr Tom Bourne; Dr Anne Prys Davies; Dr Milo Siewert, MD/DC (USA) and Sheila Leo-Siewert of the BCCM; Dr Frank Mulder and Dr Mike Evans of Park Attwood Clinic; Tom Bartram, the distinguished herbal consultant; Wendy Singer, homoeopath; Lola de Gelabert, Tad Mann and Bob Jacobs of the Wellspring Clinic; D'Anne Coburn, colonic hydrotherapist; Richard Blackwall, acupuncturist; the Bristol Cancer Help Centre, in particular Dr Rosie Thomson; Christine Steiner of the Association for New Approaches to Cancer; BACUP; Jane Martin of Cancerlink; the Breast Care and Mastectomy Association; the Woman's Health and Reproductive Rights Information Centre; the WNCC; the Cancer Research Campaign; the Imperial Cancer Research Fund; Jo and Brian Stackhouse of the Walsall Mastectomy and Breast Cancer Self Help Group, and all of their members who agreed to be 'case studies'; and the women whose stories are mentioned in this book, who all gave so unselfishly of their time and experience.

And special thanks to biologist John Stirling for his invaluable guidance and advice every step of the way.

I also wish to thank my husband, Steve, without whose support, encouragement, cooked meals and endless cups of tea this book would not have been written; and my daughter, Emily, who for one year didn't see as much of her mother as she might have liked.

Introduction

This book was written directly as a result of my own involvement with my mother's struggle with ovarian cancer – but on a broader note, it is written for all women who have a female cancer, know someone who has, or who just want to know more about the subject.

In this book the treatment options, both orthodox and alternative, are presented for the four main women's cancers: cancer of the ovaries, cancer of the cervix, cancer of the uterus and cancer of the breast. Information must be the 'key' to dealing with something as mind-blowing as a cancer diagnosis: the key to helping dissolve feelings of fear and helplessness; the key to making informed choices about treatments; the key to feeling in control of your body again; and the key to contributing to a more equal doctor-patient relationship. It is the lack of information that can sometimes kill.

There are women who may not want to use the information in this book to help them make decisions; rather, they would prefer to leave the burden of decision-making completely with their doctors. That is their right, and I respect it. But it is my hope that the majority of women reading this book will use the information gathered here to help them to get the best treatment that they possibly can, and that they will use it to stand up to any doctor or specialist who is patronising, intimidating or unsympathetic. It is a woman's right to have a say in what will happen to her own body: the cancer is in *her*, and the treatments take place *within* her.

This book is also for women who believe, like me, that there are more ways than one to fight a cancer – but orthodox medical treatments apart, they may not know where to begin to look. Alternative therapies, berated by some orthodox practitioners, have a complementary role to play in the treatment of female cancer. The major strategies for alternative cancer treatment are covered in this book, but there are some that I have not mentioned – because they are too vague, too unproved, or too 'sideline' (for example, osteopathy and chiropractic) to be of particular use to the female cancers. Some of the complementary therapies mentioned in this book may not even be available in this country, but they are mentioned because women may have heard of them and want to know more about them.

Female cancer is particularly daunting because it strikes at the heart of our femininity, sexuality and self-image, and for those reasons can be all the harder to bear. It can make you feel 'apart' from your body, or as if a part of your body has turned against you. Men have their particular male cancers (cancers of the testicles, penis and prostrate), but woman suffer more kinds of gynaecological cancer with more obvious effects.

Finally, it musn't be forgotten that it is not just the cancer patient who suffers, but her family, friends and 'carers' as well. As one female cancer patient put it, 'when a woman has cancer, it's as if the whole family comes down with the disease in their efforts to cope with it'. There is information in this book to help family, friends and carers alike to a fuller understanding of the practical and emotional problems that cancer brings in its wake so that they are better able to cope with them.

I hope that this book has succeeded in building a small bridge between the orthodox and the complementary cancer treatments, over which women can walk with confidence. I hope that I have also succeeded in creating a reference source of information that will enable women to make a package of treatments best suited to their own needs and wants.

Part One

Cancer And You

1
Introduction to Cancer

To understand more about the female cancers, you need to know exactly what cancer is. Cancer is a general term for more than one hundred diseases, characterised by an abnormal and uncontrollable growth of cells which can invade and destroy normal body tissue. Usually the division of the various kinds of cells in our bodies is orderly and controlled, but if for some reason the division process gets *out* of control, cells can develop into a lump or tumour, which can be either 'benign' or 'malignant'.

Benign

'Benign' means that the cells of the lump or tumour are not invading and destroying surrounding tissues – but if the cells continue to grow at the original site, it may put pressure on surrounding organs and cause a problem.

Malignant

A 'malignant' lump or tumour contains cells which have the ability to spread beyond the original site, which, if left un-treated, would invade and destroy surrounding tissues.

If cells *do* break away from the original (primary) tumour and spread to other parts of the body, creating a new tumour, this is known as a 'secondary' or a 'metastasis'.

THE CAUSES OF CANCER

What causes cancer is not known, but it is thought that there is no one single cause. Sir Richard Doll, Professor Emeritus of Medicine at Oxford University and one of the world's leading cancer experts, says that the development of cancer is due to three main causes: nature, nurture and luck.

'Nature' refers to our own genetic inheritance: it could be that we have inherited some abnormal chromosomes which make us more likely to get certain types of cancer; or we may have inherited a weakened ability to deal with a particular cancer. Though some cancers do seem to predominate through generations of one family, for no single cancer is there a 100 per cent risk of your inheriting the disease if a member of your family is affected. Most of the known inherited susceptibility to cancer involves making individuals more prone to other stages of the cancer-causing process, as for example by failing to repair the damage from a virus or carcinogen (cancer-causing agent) that leads to switching off genes that suppress cell growth, resulting in cells beginning to grow uncontrollably.

'Nurture' refers both to our diet and our environment. Sir Richard believes that up to 30 per cent of cancers have a dietary risk factor (that is, they could be linked to what we eat) though no individual food has so far been proved to be directly responsible for causing cancer in a human being. However, the risk is not just from our diet – the risk that our environment poses grows greater by the year.

Since the Second World War, 30,000 different chemicals have been brought into the environment, 3,000 of them as food additives alone – and some of these food additives have been proved to be carcinogenic to animals. Not enough is known about these additives, preservatives, colourings and stabilisers: how much is too much, whether they accumulate in the body and how they intermix with each other in the body. Since the war, 1,000 billion gallons of pesticide have been sprayed on English crops alone. Artificial fertilisers strip the goodness from the soil. Beef cattle and poultry are crammed full of hormones, antibiotics and growth stimulators to speed up food production. On all sides we are assaulted by environmental pollution: chemical fumes in the air we breathe, acid rain and contamination of the sea, rivers and lakes.

'Luck' depends on many factors coming together at the same time, as production of cancer depends on the body's failure to repair a whole series of DNA-damaging events. (DNA is the material of inheritance, present in every cell.) Given the number of chemicals poured into our environment in the last forty years, and the number of cigarettes smoked, it is surprising that we don't *all* have cancer. There are two principal reasons why we don't. The first is that we all have, to a greater or lesser extent, enzymes which repair damage to DNA. These enzymes are exploited when cancer patients are treated with radiotherapy. From understanding enzymes, radiotherapists know that they can give a cancer patient up to ten times or more the lethal dose of radiation if it is spread over a period of time, because 90 per cent of the damage from a dose of radiation is repaired within two hours. The other factor involved is the body's immune system, which has developed in part to eliminate pre-cancerous cells before they have mutated (changed) sufficiently to escape the 'surveillance' process (see below).

The 'luck' (or 'bad luck') factor in determining cancer development is the coincidence of several of these multiple factors – be they genetic, infectious or environmental – usually over a prolonged period of time. A few pre-disposing factors appearing together only increase your *statistical* risk of getting cancer, but you need *all* of the pre-disposing factors appearing together before a cancer can start.

THE IMMUNE SURVEILLANCE THEORY

The immune surveillance theory, shared by many orthodox and complementary therapists alike, maintains that we all have cancer cells in us from time to time, but that our healthy immune system is proficient at 'sweeping them up' before they can get up to anything. It is when our immune system becomes impaired that the random cellular aberrations get a chance, aided by other factors, to take hold and create a cancer. Dr Peter Trott, cytopathologist at the Royal Marsden Hospital, London, says, 'The immune system keeps certain fast-growing cells under control, such as epithelial cells, where most cancers originate.'

Observation of the patterns of cancer developing in patients taking immuno-suppressive drugs following heart and kidney transplants (that is, drugs which lessen the body's rejection of the new organs) or after infection with the AIDS (HIV) virus has shown that the body's immune surveillance plays an important role in cancer resistance, particularly in the pre-cancerous phase. Thereafter it is likely that the cumulative effect of small doses of numerous carcinogens over a long period of time alters the pre-cancerous cells to more lethal, invasive cancer cells. Starvation, an excess of alcohol, smoking, viruses, stress, genetic or hormonal factors, radiation and a variety of chemicals have all been shown to reduce the body's immune response. As a result of evidence from studying the effects of hypnosis on resistant wart infections of the skin, many people believe that emotional or mental trauma can also affect the immune system.

The immune surveillance theory is still just a theory which remains difficult to prove, though it has long been recognised that autopsies do reveal that a substantial number of people dying of other causes harbour areas of unsuspected, and apparently inactive, cancer.

QUESTIONS ABOUT CANCER

Cancer is a mysterious disease, sometimes escaping by changing its genetic structure to protect itself from the treatment, or by throwing up a smokescreen to avoid the immune system – but it can just as strangely disappear by itself. Cancer will not behave in the same way in each patient, even if it's the same kind of cancer. Each patient will have a different level of resistance and will react in a different way. The cure rate will be influenced by how quickly the cancer is growing, what stage it has reached at the time of diagnosis, the resistance of the patient and the treatment available and acceptable to the patient.

There is still so much about cancer that we don't yet know: why does one person get it and another not? Why does one person live with it and another die from it? Why do different cancers occur at different ages? Why can a lump be benign –

why does it grow and then stop? How many benign tumours turn malignant? These are just some of the many unanswered questions still baffling scientists. However, most important for all cancer sufferers to understand is that the diagnosis of cancer is not an automatic death sentence. As Penny Brohn, co-founder of the Bristol Cancer Help Centre, so neatly put it, 'Cancer is unpredictable: having formed, it may not grow; having grown, it may not spread; and having spread, it may not kill.' So, because of cancer's unpredictability, the attitude for anyone with cancer should be to assume 'the best' until it is obviously *not* the case.

Scientists won't find a cure for cancer until they have a better understanding of the mechanisms that control cell growth and division. If the balance between growth-stimulating messages and growth-inhibiting messages that pass between cells can be manipulated, science will be able to tackle cancer at a biological level. The secret of cancer at a genetic level is unfolding itself, but it may be another ten years before the mechanisms that trigger cancer are fully understood.

CANCER AND AGE

In the last thirty years cancer has replaced tuberculosis (TB) as the most feared disease. Those dying in their fifties and sixties from cancer now might have died in their forties and fifties a century ago from TB. The 'apparent' increase in the number of people getting cancer is due to increased lifespan: more than 80 per cent of malignant disease occurs in individuals aged forty and over, and two out of three cancers occur in people over sixty-five. Cancer is an age-related disease: if we all lived to be 150, we might *all* die of cancer!

It is thought that one in four people will contract cancer at some point in their lives, and that one in five will die from it. But orthodox doctors claim that 50 per cent of cancer patients are cured completely, and that of the other 50 per cent a substantial number experience longer survival times with a better quality of life than was possible even ten years ago. Cancer is not invariably fatal, and it must be remembered that four-fifths of all deaths in general are due to causes *other* than cancer. While the totality of cancer remains the same, the pattern of it is ever-changing; with some cancers, like stomach cancer, slowly disappearing in Western countries, and other cancers, like lung cancer, emerging more strongly.

2

You and Your Doctor

If you are diagnosed as having cancer, the relationship that you have with your GP and the cancer specialist treating you will be all-important. Most people, whether cancer patients or not, whether male or female, have a formal relationship with their doctors at best. Patients are often intimidated by their doctors' position of authority. Frequently patients have little information with which to compare the information their doctors are giving them and thus find it difficult to question or challenge their doctors.

Doctors are often viewed as larger-than-life and as having special powers over life and death that are withheld from ordinary people, so that even a normally confident person can lose her confidence in the presence of a medical professional. When a patient has cancer, wants very much to live and is afraid of dying, she will feel even more vulnerable.

Illness is such a stressful time that a woman can feel as though she has lost control – just at the point she most needs to have it. Increasingly, I'm glad to say, women are demanding a more active role in the decisions about their medical treatments, especially in the case of cancer. After all, cancer is *within* a woman, and the treatments take place within her as well. It is her body and her mental well-being that are on the line.

It is to be hoped that the 'active-passive' relationship between doctor and patient, where the doctor is 'actively' giving instructions while the patient 'passively' receives them, is giving way more and more to a relationship of mutual participation and shared responsibility. In other words the doctor helps the woman to help herself, while reinforcing her individuality and dignity.

However some women can become confused and frightened by having more information about their condition and possible treatments, and they will actually prefer to leave all decision-making in the hands of their specialist. This is their right, if they so choose. But this chapter has been written on the assumption that women actually want a more active role in the doctor/patient relationship, and a feeling of greater control over their illness. As one US cancer counsellor put it, people do not drop off their bodies at a hospital in the same way as they would drop their car off at a garage. Instead, people go to a hospital and enter into a 'contract' or covenant with the people treating them, with certain implicit assumptions about the way things should be done.

If a patient wants more information from her doctor, she should ask for it; she should also let the doctor know if she is feeling rushed, confused or intimidated. A patient has a responsibility to provide information about her physical and psychological state so that the doctor can make an accurate assessment. A doctor has a responsibility to encourage questioning by providing information in a relaxed, forthcoming manner, and in words that are easy to understand. A doctor also has a responsibility to consider the psychological needs of the patient. Research has shown that, for many patients, having information can actually reduce any pain that might be experienced during treatment, and reduce any feelings of hostility immediately *after* treatment.

DOCTORS AND COUNSELLING

In the mid-1940s, when there was only surgery and two cytotoxic drugs (ones that destroy cells) in use for cancer treatment, doctors had plenty of time to talk to their patients and to counsel them. But as soon as technological medicine took off, doctors had little time to talk to patients, and groups like the Bristol Cancer Help Centre, with its concern for the emotional and mental needs of cancer patients, were set up to fill the gap. In a society where church-going was more common, ministers and priests might have filled this gap.

As Michael Baum, Professor of Surgery at King's College

Hospital, London, admits, 'We frequently fail as communicators with our patients, and we frequently fail to fulfil the pastoral role that our clients require of us.' Many doctors are trying to return to some kind of counselling role, particularly just before and just after treatment is given, but where that is not possible support teams have sprung up in hospitals to work alongside doctors. A hospital support team consists of professionals like social workers, counsellors and nurse-counsellors.

A nurse-counsellor is a nurse who has been trained in counselling, and more and more are being trained to counsel women with female cancer. They counsel throughout a woman's treatment, and even after treatment is finished. They explain the physical and psychological implications of any treatment, and answer any personal questions which a woman may find difficult to ask her doctor. But their main role is to answer the needs that the patient herself reveals in her choice of words. Nurse-counsellors encourage women to talk, but without invading their privacy.

Sylvia Denton is a Group Senior Nurse at the Breast Unit of the Royal Marsden Hospital, London. She regards one of her jobs as helping women to make decisions. Says Sylvia, 'Some women want to be given options, while others do not. Over-informing can be cruel, and do damage – it is important to deal with a patient's individual needs. A woman should not be pushed into talking. A nurse may know more about information and practical help, but a woman knows more about how she *feels*.' Many women need not only to talk, but also to backtrack in their lives, and to discuss such deep inner feelings as 'guilt', 'divine retribution' and the fact that cancer was a 'watershed' in their lives.

Nurse-counsellors, or 'oncology nurses' as they are also called, also counsel husbands, either separately or alongside their wives. A husband or partner may have questions he wants to ask that he may be hesitant to put to his wife directly, such as how the cancer treatment will affect their sex life. A nurse-counsellor can help to bridge the communication gap between doctor and patient, or even between the patient and her husband. If a woman and her partner are told what to expect, allowed to ask questions and to air their fears and misgivings, they will both cope much better. Sylvia adds, 'A woman must still feel that she is in the driving seat and that she has been given an opportunity to become involved in the decision-making process, if possible.'

Specialist nurse-counselling has been around for only about twelve years, but many more ward sisters are now taking the course and it is hoped that soon every health district in the country will have nurse-counsellors.

Not every woman will need or want such counselling as many have their own coping mechanisms, but should you want to see a nurse-counsellor, ask at your hospital or contact your District Health Council or any of the cancer help organisations (see the list of addresses, p.276). Many of the cancer organisations, like BACUP, have counsellors you can talk to on the telephone. They can tell you how you will feel before, during and after each treatment. A number of the organisations can also put you in touch with a local self-help group, where patients and their families can meet to discuss common problems.

Many social workers are also trained counsellors who can support you at hospital or at home – ask your hospital doctor or ward sister to arrange a visit from one, if you so wish.

MACMILLAN NURSES

Macmillan nurses support and advise cancer patients at home or in hospital, and they liaise closely with hospital consultants, GPs and district nurses. They can advise on pain relief and give emotional support to patients *and* their families. (See the list of addresses, p.288.)

CHOOSING YOUR HOSPITAL/SPECIALIST

When a cancer diagnosis has been made, your best option is to be treated in a hospital that has expert staff and resources. In theory you have the right to be treated in a hospital of your choice, where there is a specialist (oncologist) in your kind of cancer. If you have the name of a specialist, check that he/she works in a hospital near you, and how long the waiting list is.

Whoever you choose, you may want to know in advance what his/her views are on various treatments. You may also want to know what kind of aftercare is on offer from the hospital of your choice, such as whether there is a hospital 'patient group' for your kind of cancer.

The Social Services department of your hospital can advise you about any local organisations that offer help to cancer patients and their families, which may include financial aid and transport to and from the hospital.

TALKING TO YOUR SPECIALIST

When you first see your specialist, prepare a list of questions to ask him. Bring a relative or friend with you, not only to give you the extra confidence to ask the questions, but also to help you to remember the answers! If at all possible, bring a tiny, hand-sized tape recorder with you, and tape the entire conversation. That way, you won't forget anything. It is surprising how much you can forget when you are feeling anxious or confused.

Here are some suggestions for questions:

- What treatments are possible?
- Which treatments do you recommend, and why?
- What is the aim of each treatment, and how successful do you think it will be?
- How long before I know if the treatment is achieving its aim?
- What are the chances of cure/control/pain relief?
- Are there any risks involved?
- What will the side effects be?
- What will happen if I don't have the treatments that you suggest?
- When does treatment finish?
- How often will I need medical check-ups after treatment?
- What should I tell my relatives and friends?

If you were thinking of taking complementary treatments either before or alongside orthodox treatments, you could ask:

- If I wanted to try other types of treatment before the ones that you recommend, how much time would I have before the cancer grew or started to spread? (The doctor won't be able to give you an exact idea, but an estimate will do.)

- How would you feel if I wanted to take complementary therapies alongside orthodox treatment?

Don't be put off if the specialist is hostile or unreceptive to this last question. If you feel strongly about taking both kinds of treatments together in order to get the best of both worlds, you may even want to switch to a more sympathetic specialist, or at least convince your specialist to keep an open mind for a while. Most specialists, however, would not take a negative view of such an approach, as alternative therapies used in a complementary way *enhance* orthodox treatments rather than interfere or hinder them. Remember that you have a right to the kind of treatment that *you* want!

Do not let the doctor intimidate or rush you; don't feel stupid if you need information repeated even more than once, or explained in a different way. It is the doctor's responsibility to persevere until you understand. Doctors look for clues to help them decide how much a patient wants to know all at once – that is why, if you do not ask for information, you may be given only what is necessary.

Never be rushed or pressurised into a decision before understanding everything that is involved. In fact, take the time to find out all the advantages and disadvantages of each possible treatment. Even if you haven't had a cancer diagnosis, but are worried that one day you might have, it is extremely helpful to think through what kind of treatment you would like and how you would deal with it, while you are still clear-headed and objective. What would you need in the way of help at home, or cover on your job, for instance?

In fact, if you want a second, third or fourth opinion, that is your right too – your specialist won't mind referring you on, as he/she is used to dealing with this kind of request. Or you could be referred to someone else through your GP. You may want to get at least *one* different opinion before embarking on the treatment which your specialist proposes, particularly to confirm the diagnosis and the line of treatment. This also applies to any doubts you may have about the accuracy of tests done: it is a patient's right to be able to ask for a second test to be done in a different hospital.

Discuss all possible options about surgery beforehand with the specialist, and remember that no operation or procedure will be done without your consent. After any surgery, ask the surgeon or doctor to make up a list of any important post-surgery care that you could take home with you, and go over it with him/her step by step. In the end, all decisions are yours, because apart from it being *your* body and *your* health, you are the only one who knows what you are prepared to go through for possible recovery. What you should aim to do is to take a more active role in your recovery. Somewhere there exists a compromise between accepting help and becoming a part of the decision-making process.

Remember that the specialist is not God; he/she cannot tell you exactly how you will react to each treatment, or how long you will live. All the specialist can do is give you general information about what the 'average' patient can expect, and the best and worst that can happen on the basis of his/her experience and the statistics. And once in hospital, don't compare your treatment programme with another woman's: it could well be different from yours, as the same cancer can affect two people differently. Also, she may have had to come to a different agreement about treatment with her therapist.

Changing your hospital doctor

If you are unhappy with your hospital doctor, and you feel that you have already given him/her a fair chance, you can ask your GP to refer you to a different doctor at a different hospital – to someone they know, you know, or someone recommended by one of the cancer help organisations. Keep in mind, though, that a change could mean a longer, more expensive journey or delays in treatment.

CLINICAL TRIALS

With so many different combinations of treatments available, the running of clinical trials to decide their worth is very important. If your doctor or specialist wants to enter you into a clinical trial to test the benefit of a treatment, make sure that you know what the choice is: in other words, what will your group be testing, and what will the other group be testing? What are the other options for you? Before giving your consent, ask the doctor all about the testing procedure, its purpose, risks and side effects, and its advantages/disadvantages over other forms of treatment for you. You must know what the other choices are, and that none of them is known to be any better than what you will be receiving.

You are entitled to know if a procedure is experimental or un-proven. Sometimes a woman is randomly appointed to a particular treatment group by computer, and the doctor running the trial has not made this clear. Read the 'informed consent' form carefully, and ask for clarification of terms where needed. This form mentions any drug therapy or radiotherapy treatment which may be included in the trial, and makes clear the patient's rights.

You can consult with others before making a decision, and you can withdraw from a trial at any stage and still be entitled to treatment from the same consultant. Any treatment that is clearly not helping you should be stopped, and any changes in the research treatment should only be agreed to if they are beneficial to you.

PAIN CONTROL

No patient needs to suffer with pain: most cancers do not cause pain unless they are pressing on a nerve, and even in a late-stage cancer, pain is not inevitable. There may be some pain after a treatment like surgery, while cut tissues are healing. The level of pain that an individual experiences is a measure of how her body chemicals are reacting to the situation, so everyone will experience pain differently, and it is no measure of 'bravery' or the lack of it if one woman feels less or more pain than another. Pain can be controlled without drugs through acupuncture or hypnosis, or through a variety of orthodox painkillers, ranging from aspirin, paracetamol and distalgesic, through the codeine preparations, to the narcotics, which can be prescribed only by a doctor.

Though a small number of patients who need to use narcotics

may develop dependency, if the cause of the pain is eliminated it is almost unknown for a patient to be left with a permanent addiction problem. As narcotics are by far and away the best painkillers, doctors stress that the so-called 'fear of addiction' shouldn't put patients off using narcotic drugs when they are needed. The major side effects are drowsiness, nausea, constipation and sometimes vomiting, though it is usually possible to find ways around these symptoms, which are temporary and stop occurring when the body has adjusted to the drugs.

As a last resort if pain is severe and restricted to one area, there is the 'nerve block', where a hospital anaesthethist gives an injection to block off pain signals – but this is rarely used.

Avoid aspirin preparations if you are on chemotherapy, as they damage blood platelets (cells which help the blood to clot).

It is best not to anticipate pain, but to keep yourself busy with some engrossing activity. Norman Cousins, a former writer and senior lecturer in medicine at the University of California, fought off the pain of his late-stage cancer with video movies of the Marx brothers and other comedy shows. The laughter these shows engendered produced an anaesthetic effect in his body, by helping to release the body's own endorphins – morphine-like substances produced naturally in the brain that help lessen pain.

3

Cancer and You

REACTIONS TO CANCER

A diagnosis of cancer brings an often overwhelming variety of feelings and emotions to the surface in most people. How one woman reacts is different from the way that another might react – there is no right or wrong way to feel. Remember that all feelings are just a way of coming to terms with the illness.

Shock is normally the first feeling; a kind of 'numbness' where everything seems slightly unreal. Information just doesn't sink in, so you keep asking the same questions over and over again. Don't worry – this is quite a normal reaction.

Anger may be another immediate reaction: 'Why me?'; 'Why Now?'; 'It's not fair' and so on. You may feel like railing at your doctor, your family and friends, and at God. You may be angry at that part of your body which you feel has betrayed you. This is another perfectly normal reaction that merely shows how upset you are about your illness, and your family and friends shouldn't take it personally – your doctor certainly won't!

Anger needs to be expressed, because bottled up it can eat away at you – but when let out, it can give you the energy to take positive action. Strangely enough, most people don't get angry when they receive the bad news. Yet perhaps more people should, because research shows that angry people are highly motivated to help themselves fight against the disease, and fare better in the long run.

Denial. For some patients, the shock can be so great that they deny that they have cancer. This may just be a disguised cry for help, a natural reaction to the fear of not being able to cope. These patients may benefit from counselling from someone such as a cancer-trained nurse. Ironically, some degree of denial – hearing what you want to hear, but disregarding the rest – may be the best coping mechanism for some patients, and may help them to sail through treatments with few problems. If family and friends suspect this to be the case, they should tread gently.

Guilt. After the initial shock has subsided, many patients start blaming themselves: 'If only I hadn't done/said/felt . . .' This is normal too, as doctors don't know what causes cancer, so the sufferer naturally picks an easy target – herself. This isn't a healthy state of affairs because, cigarette smoking apart, there is rarely any truth to it. It takes the coming together of many factors at the same time to cause a cancer. Instead of blaming yourself, it is much better to get yourself into a fighting frame of mind, which makes you determined to conquer the disease.

Withdrawal. Some people may withdraw into themselves for a while, to mull over the implications and ramifications of their illness and to sort out their feelings. This again is normal, but if it goes on for too long, a friend or family member should arrange for some counselling.

Resentment. It may be hard for a cancer patient *not* to resent everyone else's apparent good health when she has been struck down herself. The spouse or 'carer' may feel resentment too, because their life has been so quickly and drastically altered. It helps to get resentment out in the open, so that it can blow away without doing any lasting damage, rather than let it lie and fester.

Fear. Every woman given a cancer diagnosis will be afraid and uncertain about what is going to happen to her in the immediate present in the form of treatments, and about what her long-term chances are. Although the idea of dying is one that everyone must come to terms with sooner or later, a cancer diagnosis makes death appear more immediate, and having cancer is a constant reminder of one's own fragile mortality. If thoughts or fears about dying become overwhelming, a woman could seek out a religious leader (if she followed a particular religion), a counsellor or a psychotherapist. Sometimes just bringing out such fears into the open with a loved one can be enough. Fear of the *unknown* can be allayed by collecting as much information as possible.

There may also be a fear of pain to come, but with many cancers there is little or no pain, and with today's modern pain-killing drugs or the use of acupuncture, no one should have to suffer pain. (See p.16 and Chapter 13.)

Grief and Loss. For women who need to have surgery there will be a deep feeling of loss for the part of the body that has been removed and a mourning for that loss. Particularly with a female cancer, a woman may be mourning the loss of part of her female identity, or of her fertility. Grief, like anger, should never be bottled up: once released, it will dissipate with time, but bottling it up could prolong it indefinitely.

The process of grieving should never be hurried along by well-meaning family and friends. No woman should have to listen to the mindless platitudes of 'Chin up' or 'Pull yourself together'. Each woman needs her own grieving period, the length of which varies from person to person. Again, professional counselling can help, particularly if grieving begins adversely to affect a woman's health. One thing that counselling can do is to help a woman explore her feelings about herself and her cancer – the emotional aspect of cancer should never be overlooked.

FAMILY AND FRIENDS

Family and friends can be just as devastated by a cancer diagnosis, and some may need professional counselling help in order to cope. They may well feel shut out and confused by your reactions and feelings if you have cancer, and may not know what to do or say. It will be up to you to tell them what you need in the way of emotional and practical support. Don't try to handle cancer all by yourself, because then everyone will lose: you will lose the opportunity to express how you feel, and your family and friends will lose the opportunity of truly understanding what your needs and problems are.

If you feel that you are not getting enough sympathy from your family, perhaps you are not sending out the right signals. Remember that you are entitled to sympathy and support, so don't be shy of asking for it! If you expect others to 'guess' how you are feeling, you will only become angry with them for their insensitivity if they get it wrong.

Talking to children

Telling any children in the family about your cancer can be difficult, but an open, honest approach is always best. Listen to their fears and, as children are prone to blame themselves, reassure them that your cancer is not their fault. Watch for any changes in their behaviour: this will be their own way of expressing their feelings. Start with a very simple explanation if the children are young, and give out more information as their age and maturity demands.

Your partner

A partner may feel rejected, especially if you have gone off sex or don't want to be touched after a cancer treatment, when in fact it may be *you* who feels 'rejectable' and lacking in confidence. A husband may not be touching his wife for fear of hurting her, but because he hasn't said this, the wife feels doubly rejected. It is all down to a lack of communication, and consequent misunderstanding. Try to keep the channels of communication open between you both, no matter how hurt and mixed up you are feeling. It might not hurt to remind a partner that cancer is not 'catching', even when making love.

Cancer is an illness that can change us physically, altering our self-image and perhaps changing our perception of what we find pleasurable in love-making. The intimacy between two people can be temporarily shaken by cancer, but it should not be permanently shaken. Many couples are brought even closer together by the cancer experience, particularly if it is shared from the start. Some relationships may not survive, but when this happens, there is usually a history of problems in the relationship.

A relationship is based on many things besides physical attraction: friendship, shared experiences, mutual trust, a similar outlook and life goals, similar interests and, of course, mutual love. If cancer has rocked the foundations of a relationship, seek out counselling for the two of you straight away. The more the two of you can talk about your fears and anxieties, the better able you will be to resolve them.

PHYSICAL PROBLEMS

There can be physical problems with love-making soon after surgery or radiotherapy. Radiotherapy to the vagina or cervix can result in scarred tissue that has lost some elasticity. The production of natural secretions could also be affected, resulting in decreased lubrication.

But having sex as soon after treatment as you feel like it (with the consent of your doctor) can actually improve the situation by helping to keep the tissues stretched. Using one, then eventually two or more fingers gently to stretch the vagina will help; or you can obtain a vaginal dilator through your GP or chemist. Using a lubricant like KY Jelly or changing your position during sex to avoid painful areas will also help.

It will be about a six-week wait after a hysterectomy before sex is possible. If you are pre-menopausal it may take longer to sort out all of your emotions, which will be aggravated by the sudden drop in hormone levels. Some women will also take a while to adjust to a breast scar – many women are afraid to let their partner see it. This is where a little tender loving care on the part of the spouse comes into its own. It often helps if the couple start looking at the breast scar together in hospital, as it then won't be such a big deal when the woman returns home.

The removal of ovaries brings on an early menopause, with hot flushes, dry skin, vaginal dryness, and a decrease in sexual desire. The loss of sex drive can also occur during chemo-therapy. Sexual desire usually returns when you are feeling more yourself, but speak to your doctor about the possibility of hormone replacement therapy, and use KY Jelly for any vaginal dryness.

Sometimes the loss of sex drive occurs even before a cancer diagnosis. Don't let sexual problems continue; contact an organisation like RELATE, which specialises in sexual counselling (see the list of addresses, p. 285). Some women are not told when to resume sex, mainly because their doctor forgets to tell them, so don't be afraid to *ask*.

TALKING TO OTHERS

Allow yourself to *express* your feelings: contrary to what you might think, expressing feelings doesn't mean that you will lose control over them; rather, it allows you to *stay* in control of them. Be open with your feelings and fears, and talk to others: to your spouse, family, friends, doctors, nurses and other cancer patients.

Dr Vicky Clement-Jones, who formed BACUP (British Association of Cancer United Patients and their families and friends – see page 277), was a Senior Registrar in the Department of Endocrinology at St Bartholomew's Hospital in London, and aged thirty-two, when it was discovered that she had advanced ovarian cancer. At first she was given a private room of her own to match her doctor status; but later she was moved into a gynaecological ward, where she finally met another ovarian cancer patient. In an article in the *British Medical Journal* in October 1985, Vicky wrote: 'We shared our experiences of chemotherapy, anticipatory vomiting, the trauma of repeated venopuncture with ever-vanishing veins, the loss of child-bearing and the onset of menopausal hot flushes, and in this way we supported each other through these difficult times. Through this experience, I realised that other patients could give me something unique which I could not obtain from my doctors, or nurses, however caring.'

Pauline Young, another ovarian cancer patient, told me that women with cancer should 'talk things out, with anyone – the more you do it, the more it helps you.' It was through talking to her friends at work that she made a few discoveries of her own. Says Pauline, 'People get the wrong idea about cancer. My friends could not believe that you could have cancer and look so well on it, that you could have cancer and live longer than six months, or that there were actually treatments that *worked* for cancer.'

FEELINGS AFTER TREATMENT

Ironically, some women can feel more depressed *after* cancer treatments are over, when they are on the road to recovery and

back to their everyday lives. It is not hard to understand why:
for months, perhaps years, the patient has been cocooned in
medical attention and perhaps fussed over by family and
friends. Re-channelling energy from merely 'surviving' to
planning a future again takes time and can be a big adjustment
to make.

At this point, joining a cancer self-help group (see the list of
addresses, p.276) can be an extremely positive move. There you
will meet other patients who feel the same way as you do, and
sharing your experiences can speed along recovery. In fact the
benefits are even greater if you join such a group as soon as you
are given a cancer diagnosis: learning ways to cope physically
and emotionally with problems that arise during treatments,
and sharing the camaraderie and support of fellow patients can
be a great morale-booster.

THE CANCER PERSONALITY

Many people wonder whether there is such a thing as a 'cancer
personality', a specific type of person who is prone to cancer.
There is some evidence to suggest that there might be. As far
back as the second century AD, Galen observed that 'melan-
cholic women were more prone to breast cancer than their
sanguine sisters'. Psychological disturbances create chemical
changes in the body which can actually be measured by modern
science.

Lawrence Le Shan, a twentieth-century American psychologist, has put together a profile of the 'cancer personality', after
interviewing thousands of cancer patients and their families
over a period of ten years. He also studied the case notes of
thousands of other cancer patients. His 'cancer personality'
always suffered traumatic childhood events, which lead to the
following characteristics:

- A poor self-image.
- A general feeling of inadequacy which developed early in life.
- An inability to express emotions.
- Lack of an outlet for creative energy.
- A sense of self-defeat about his/her own endeavours.

However, other research shows that 30 per cent of cancer patients do not have any of the aforementioned characteristics, so we must be careful not to be too quick to pin the 'cancer personality' label on every cancer patient (or indeed on every healthy person) who suffered a traumatic childhood or who simply appears meek, quiet or introverted.

But, to follow Lawrence Le Shan's research for a moment, he discovered that all the cancer patients he had studied had experienced the loss of an important relationship, followed by depression. To test his hypothesis, a colleague of Le Shan's mixed the case histories of cancer patients in with the case histories of other patients – and Le Shan was able to pick out 80 per cent of the cancer patients.

The Bristol Cancer Help Centre seems to confirm Le Shan's findings with the following profile of their 'average' cancer patient:

- A 'do-gooder'; a kind, nice person in a caring profession who has trouble expressing negative emotions, especially in his/her own defence; someone who finds it difficult to say 'no', while putting other people's needs ahead of their own. In fact, many of these people are extremely angry and frustrated inside, but allow themselves no outlet for it. If you add a low self-image to this picture, you will understand why some visitors to the Bristol Cancer Help Centre have trouble doing visualisation (see page 251), as they don't really believe they are worth saving!

Women seem to fit more easily into this profile, and it would be true to say that more women have been trained from childhood to believe that they are loved not for themselves but for what they *do* – in other words, affection from others comes only as a reward for good deeds. Along with this comes a fear of saying 'no' in case this would lead to others withdrawing their affection. And so often a 'cancer personality' would continue to be nice, even when they didn't want to be.

According to these cancer profiles, if a woman loses a central relationship through death, divorce or separation, it is thought to affect her more strongly as she is more accustomed to defining herself in terms of others ('John's wife', 'Mary's mother') and seeing herself as an appendage rather than as an autonomous being.

One doctor who works in the field of complementary medi-cine has his own theories about why some of his female patients have cancer. Although he acknowledges that his theories certainly do not apply to every case of female cancer he has seen, a few themes kept recurring:

- Women with 'unused reproductive processes' – that is, women who had never had children and secretly wanted them.
- Women with deep sexual problems that had never been worked out.
- Women with unresolved *life* problems: for instance, a woman who had never been accepted as a complete person by her husband.
- Women who were 'innocents', with few defences against other people.

Even orthodox doctors have noticed similarities in patients with a particular kind of cancer. One doctor who works with ovarian cancer patients was struck by the fact that many of his patients tended to be 'gentle, uncomplaining, accepting, introverted types'. But he was quick to add that perhaps there were other common denominators in an ovarian cancer group that rose above personality, such as the age of the woman or not having had any children.

If the 'personality factor' ever becomes more firmly proven, it could be used only to identify women at risk – it could never work as a preventative, for the simple reason that personality is difficult to change.

It is necessary to tread warily with such generalisations, but sometimes the woman herself recognises what she believes to be the emotional root of her cancer. This is not to say that all or most cancers have emotional origins: straightforward physical causes seem more relevant for many other women. We must be careful about categorising ourselves or others in such a way, as it can lead to self-blame, guilt and putting ourselves firmly back in the 'victim' role.

Any therapist who insists to you that your cancer has solely a deep emotional or spiritual problem as its main cause should be viewed with some scepticism. A woman with cancer has enough on her plate without piling on more guilt and self-recrimination

– and even if she *does* identify her illness with an underlying emotional problem, she should use that knowledge positively, to change those aspects of her life which are unsatisfactory, rather than to blame herself further.

STRESS

Stress has been shown to affect the immune system, but there isn't yet a direct link between stress and cancer – at the very most, stress is only a co-factor, not a *cause*, of cancer. Rats and mice are more likely to develop tumours if they are stressed, but people are different from rats and mice, and what stresses one person doesn't necessarily stress another – except perhaps the major traumas of death of a loved one, divorce or separation, and loss of a job. Remarks biologist John Stirling, 'If stress was a cause of cancer, none of us would have got past childhood. Stressful events happen just as often to people who don't develop cancer as to those who *do*.'

And yet there is some chemical basis for the stress/cancer link. Research in the USA on medical students showed changes in the number of 'killer' cells in their immune system around a stressful event like studying for an exam. Stress hormones that build up in the bloodstream can interfere with the production of T-lymphocytes (a type of white blood cell), and upset delicate chemical balances in the immune system. Stress affects the endocrine glands like the thyroid, which is the glandular link between the brain and the reproductive organs. The thyroid can be stimulated or inhibited by emotional upsets, which in turn affect the circulation, respiration, tissue growth and repair.

However, mental and emotional stress are not automatic precursors to cancer. Stress may affect the immune system, as it affects certain physical processes, but it is not yet clear *how*. The mystery will not be fully unravelled until we learn more about the way the neuro-endocrine system controls the immune system. Can stress lower the immune system by, say, affecting hormone levels and thus allowing cancer cells to grow? Can sheer determination, such as positive visualisation (see p.251), help the immune system destroy cancer cells? No one yet knows.

We can be stressed on a *physical* level without even realising it by such things in our environment as certain types of artificial lighting, cosmic radiation and the background radiation given off by electrical appliances and office equipment.

There is some evidence to suggest that if one partner of a couple gets cancer, the other is more likely to develop it. Has this to do with shared environmental factors and/or psychological stress? Perhaps our immune system does not function as well when we are experiencing fear, depression and frustration.

Stress in itself can be less important than the way in which we *handle* it – in other words, how we actually cope when reacting to outside challenges. Interestingly enough, cancer levels dropped during the Second World War (a very stressful time for everyone concerned) and rose again afterwards. One reason could have been a diet lower in fats and sugar, and hence in calories, but another reason could have been that the stress we create for ourselves wreaks more internal havoc than the stress perceived as coming from an outside source.

If we know how to recover from stress so that stress hormones don't build up in the bloodstream, we can avoid doing any damage to our immune system. The problem is when we stay 'stressed' for long periods of time – and for some people a perpetually stressed state is normal. Stressful events in your early life can 'use up' your stress 'tolerance' levels, so that you become less able to cope with stress efficiently when you are older. Activities like exercise, relaxation, meditation, an absorbing hobby, creative outlet or a pleasurable pursuit, can defuse stress before it gets a long-term hold. A healthy, well-adjusted person will not stay stressed forever: when the stress is passed, the body returns to normal.

Studies on stress and cancer patients are by nature inconclusive, as there is no way to separate the stress created by the cancer *itself*. And what is often overlooked is that the chemical reactions taking place in the body as a result of the cancer's activities can also affect moods directly. As John Stirling remarks, 'The formation of tumours produces toxic residues which in themselves can alter blood chemistry and create depression. After a tumour is removed, patients often feel better and brighter, and part of this is due to their blood chemistry improving.'

A POSITIVE ATTITUDE

If stress *does* have a negative effect on the immune system, can cultivating a 'positive' attitude have a positive effect? A study carried out in 1982 by psychologist Stephen Green at King's College Hospital looked at the value of psychotherapy for patients with breast cancer: the patients who did the best had a strong, hostile drive without the loss of emotional control – in other words, the opposite of a 'hopeless' reaction. Those with a fighting spirit lived twice as long as those who just 'gave in'. So *does* optimism stimulate the immune system?

Therapists in complementary medicine believe that positive feelings can arrest or even reverse cancer growth. If the mind is charged with positive energy, the theory goes, the body will respond to the mind's overwhelming desire for good health by getting rid of the cancer (see p.251). We still do not fully understand the interplay of mind and body, but many doctors and therapists alike believe that the link exists, and that this link just needs to be discovered.

It is interesting to note also that orthodox doctors believe the reverse to be true: that you can go downhill fast, and even bring about your early demise through a negative attitude. As one doctor puts it, when patients are given limited horizons, they tend to limit their expectations as well.

Carl Simonton, the cancer oncologist who developed the idea of 'positive visualisation' (see p.251), claims that the shared factor in cases of spontaneous remission of cancer is a positive attitude, although this is theory, not 'proven fact'. Some therapists in complementary medicine would go even further and say that spontaneous remissions seem to be preceded by a new outlook and an acceptance of the self's responsibility for healing and recovery.

Having a negative attitude in itself will not make you susceptible to cancer: the number of 'depressives' who get cancer is not very high. Having a negative attitude after cancer is diagnosed is understandable, but as there appears to be some link between our feelings and our immune system, this is one thing that cancer patients should strive to avoid. Who knows? – a positive attitude may make that vital bit of difference, and it will undoubtedly improve the quality of a patient's life. Also, it is one more constructive thing that a woman can do for herself, perhaps for the first time in her life. And if it can ever be proved that a positive emotional attitude can stimulate the body's immune system, perhaps one day we will see (as Dr Stephen Green believes we will) the development of methods of psychological intervention that will be used alongside standard cancer treatments not only to improve the quality of life, but also in some cases even to lengthen survival time.

Part Two
Orthodox Treatments

4

The Orthodox Approach to the Four Women's Cancers

Over 120,000 new cases of cancer occur in women in the UK every year; at any one time, there are over 700,000 women alive who have had a cancer diagnosis. One in five women die of cancer: a total of 71,000 every year. Apart from the major cancers that are shared between the sexes (skin, lung, colon and stomach cancers), women face an added cancer risk from their own sexual and reproductive organs: namely, ovaries, cervix, uterus and breast. These are the four main female cancers, although there are a few other, quite rare ones which will be mentioned later.

Both orthodox doctors and complementary therapists view cancer as an uncontrollable mass of growing cells, which may eventually kill the patient by using up nutrients, releasing toxins and crowding the vital organs. Orthodox treatments for the four female cancers, by which is meant what Western science has to offer, consists of surgery, radiotherapy, chemotherapy and hormone therapy.

FIVE-YEAR SURVIVAL RATES

Before going into an explanation of approaches to the four cancers, I would like first to explain the orthodox definition of successful treatment and the orthodox approach to survival rates.

Success of orthodox treatments is measured at three levels: first, in terms of the doctor's ability to render the patient free of cancer symptoms; second, in terms of the doctor's ability to clear the patient of the physical evidence of cancer; and third, in terms of *survival*. Because some cancers may recur five, ten or even fifteen years after treatment finishes, and some patients who have had one cancer develop a second, most doctors treating cancer patients follow them indefinitely to be sure of the success of their treatments.

Orthodox doctors often speak of a five-year survival rate, which means how many patients are alive five years after *primary* treatment (usually surgery) is given. This means that cancer patients aim to get through five years without having a relapse (recurrence) – after five years they are unlikely to have a relapse, although there is a small chance with breast cancer. David Oram, gynaecological surgeon at the London Hospital, says: 'In the majority of cancers, if a cancer is going to relapse, it will do so within the first two years after diagnosis.'

LIFE EXPECTANCY

Although doctors say that they never predict life-expectancy for an individual patient, they may sometimes talk about a 'median' life-expectancy: for example, a six-month median life-expectancy means that half the patients in the same cancer group will be alive in six months. This is *not* the same as applying it to an individual patient, however. If pressed by a patient or her relatives, a doctor may talk about 'median' life-expectancy, but this is *not* the same as telling you how long you have to live. No doctor can do that and, ethically speaking, most wouldn't try. Doctors are not gods and do not possess a crystal ball – the human body is a remarkable thing, and sometimes patients go on to defy all the medical odds and even recover when recovery wasn't part of the medical picture. Cancers can go into a remission all by themselves, sometimes even without treatment, and some can remain in a body in a controlled, quiet state for many years, or even until the patient dies from some other cause. What doctors *can* tell, though, is when a patient is 'terminal' – that is, when he/she only has a few days left to live.

THE TREATMENT OPTIONS

Surgery aims to cut out the cancer cells, radiotherapy to burn them, chemotherapy to poison them and hormone therapy to cut off their growth messages. Orthodox treatments are used in a carefully planned sequence of treatments, depending on the type, size, stage and spread of a tumour, and the age and general health of a patient. They must be used with care so as not to damage the patient's immune system, which has to get rid of the last bits of cancer by itself. Orthodox treatments succeed to varying degrees with different cancers, and in the cases where a cure is not possible they can at least alleviate symptoms and improve the quality of the remaining years of life.

SURGERY

Surgery is usually the first line of attack on a tumour. Its aim is to remove every bit of cancer that can be seen or reached in an operation without harming the vital organs. The visible growth as well as a wide margin of surrounding normal tissue is removed. The majority of female cancers will require some degree of surgery, even if only a lumpectomy for breast cancer or a cone biopsy for cervical cancer. (The various surgical procedures for each of the female cancers is described in the relevant chapters.)

Surgery is the most widespread and successful of the orthodox techniques for tumours that haven't spread – but there is a fine balance to be maintained between removing too little of the cancer and therefore risking spread, and removing too much healthy tissue and so causing complications. Nobody can be sure of the outcome. It is a myth that oxygen entering the body during surgery can speed up the growth of a cancer – actually, cancer thrives on low oxygen. If cancer spread *does* occur after surgery, it could be that either the spread took place beforehand and was not detected by any of the routine screening procedures or that some cancer cells broke loose during the tumour removal.

The additional factor could be that surgery, or the actual

Women's Cancers

anaesthetic drug used in surgery, suppresses the immune system, and allows minute forms of rapidly developing cells to gain a foothold in the scar tissue, which is vulnerable to cancer.

RADIOTHERAPY

Radiotherapy, or radiation therapy, aims to destroy cancer with radiation such as X-rays, cobalt or gamma rays. These damage the cancer cells' genetic material so that they are unable to divide. It is used to shrink or destroy localised areas of cancerous tumours, or is used before and/or after an operation to increase the chances of a successful cure, as in breast cancer. Radiotherapy does this by reducing the risk that any cancer cells 'split' at the time of surgery might take root. It can also be used following surgery when there has been secondary spread – it is particularly good for bone secondaries and for cancers like breast cancer, where the growth has broken through the skin. It is also used to relieve pain in advanced stages of cancer. In the last ten years there have been improvements in radiotherapy, making it quicker and safer.

Radioactive implants (like radioactive gold, which emits alpha particles) are sometimes used for breast, cervical and uterine cancers. These implants give a large dose of radio-activity directly to the cancer, while giving very little radio-activity to the surrounding tissue. For some cancers, radiotherapy is used without any other treatment and is curative; while for other cancers, even though the chance of a cure is slight, it slows down the growth and relieves symptoms. It works best on precisely defined tumours, or in cases where it is best not to remove the organ being treated, such as the cervix.

Radiotherapy treatment

Before radiotherapy treatment, preliminary X-rays of the patient's cancer are taken and marks are put on the skin to show the radiographer the exact place to direct the rays. The machines used for treatment are usually 'linear accelerators' – during treatment the patient lies on a couch while the machine is positioned carefully over the pre-drawn marks. The radiotherapist leaves the room before the machine is switched on, to protect herself from accumulated doses of radiation she might otherwise receive by remaining in the room. The treatment is quite painless and lasts only a few minutes; it is given on an outpatient basis for three to six weeks at a time, with from one to five sessions a week, with a rest at weekends. The length of your overall treatment depends on the type and size of your cancer.

During treatment you must keep the area of skin treated as dry as possible, to prevent the skin from becoming red and sore. Drink lots of fluids, get as much rest as you can and supplement meals with high-calorie (replacement meal) drinks if your appetite is poor. Don't worry; radiotherapy does not make you radioactive, so you can be with others over your treatment period.

Radiotherapy aims to give as high a dose of radiation as possible to a tumour without damaging the normal tissue around it – as every tissue has a different tolerance level. Normal cells *do* get damaged as well, although the body can repair 90 per cent of radiation damage in under three hours. The body can do this even after a large dose, which explains why survivors of major radioactive accidents do not all die of cancer.

Side effects of radiotherapy

There can be side effects to radiotherapy, and there are two different types: acute and chronic.

Acute side effects start early and are usually short-lived and disappear within three to eight weeks after stopping treatment, usually when you are recovering at home. Side effects can consist of skin soreness, nausea, diarrhoea, fatigue and burning sensation when passing urine. Diarrhoea is more applicable when the *lower* part of the abdomen is being irradiated. Sore skin can be treated with a special cream which will be given to you, and drugs can be given to combat any sickness or diarrhoea. The most acute side effect is vomiting, which may occur in some patients within a few hours of treatment if the stomach is being irradiated. Most other side effects build up over the period of treatment and peak two to three weeks after its completion.

Chronic side effects are delayed, and more serious. Whereas acute radiation side effects are less troublesome than those of acute chemotherapy, *chronic* radiation side effects are worse than those of chronic chemotherapy. Depending on the area irradiated, blood vessels or the bladder opening or the bowels could narrow, causing discomfort which may require an operation (in the case of bladder and bowels) in order to gain relief. The possibility of the bladder or bowels being affected arises only when the abdomen is irradiated and can affect 5 to 25 per cent of patients having abdominal radiotherapy, depending on the dose, which is why doctors do not like irradiating this area. The abdomen, unlike some other parts of the body, has a very low tolerance to radiotherapy.

It is interesting to note that, with short exposure and low doses, radiation can be used as a diagnostic tool; while with short exposure and higher doses, it is a therapeutic treatment – but that in chronic low doses, over long periods of time, it can contribute to causing cancer. The most clear-cut evidence of this has come from careful follow-up of survivors of the atomic bombs dropped on the Japanese cities of Hiroshima and Nagasaki during the Second World War – though even today, more than fifty years later, the majority of the surviving individuals have not developed cancer, perhaps reflecting the fact that they have particularly good DNA repair mechanisms.

Cosmic radiation is thought to be one of the carcinogens that we are exposed to daily, and ultraviolet radiation from the sun can cause skin cancer. It is known that too many X-rays of the body over a lifetime can lead to a cancer.

Radiation is measured in micro sieverts: one micro sievert is equal to one-tenth of your average dose from a single chest X-ray. The level of radiation that you will receive during radiotherapy will vary, depending on what organ is being treated and the purpose of the treatment. If you are being treated with a high dose, it will be given over a shorter period of time in order to reduce the toxicity and to cut down on delayed symptoms. In some centres, research is being done to see if the toxicity and delayed symptoms of higher doses can be avoided – this involves giving radiotherapy three times a day in lower doses rather than once a day in a higher dose. Before you start your treatment, you should ask your radiotherapist and the planning radiographer to explain to you the schedule and the dosage that you will be receiving.

CHEMOTHERAPY

Just as for some cancers surgery or radiotherapy is the treatment of choice, so there are others, particularly in young people, where chemotherapy is the treatment of choice to achieve a 'cure'. Chemotherapy ('chemo') may be used when radiotherapy is not possible, as when the cancer is too widespread or there are secondaries present – in these circumstances, chemo can still relieve symptoms. Chemotherapy involves using cytotoxic ('cell poisoning') drugs which combine with and then damage the genetic material (DNA) of cancer cells so that they can't divide properly. Some normal cells are affected too, and the art of chemotherapy, according to oncologist Tim Oliver, is to poison the person 'just to the limit of the patient's tolerance, on the basis that the cancer cell has less efficient DNA repair systems than normal cells'.

Chemotherapy came into its own as a result of an accident during the Second World War when the Germans blew up an Allied ship loaded with poisonous mustard gas. The gas killed many soldiers by destroying their bone marrow so that they bled, became anaemic and developed infections. Scientists reasoned that if it had such a dramatic effect on the most rapidly dividing cells in the body (that is, bone marrow cells), it might also have the same effect on cancer cells. The first patients selected for chemotherapy treatment were those with cancers arising in blood cells (red blood cells are produced in the bone marrow). These patients suffering from Hodgkin's disease or leukaemia experienced amazing, if short-lived, remissions. Scientists then began to search for other substances that could damage the genetic material of cells so that they couldn't divide properly – and this work laid the foundations of modern chemotherapy.

Chemotherapy can be given orally, but it is usually given intravenously (that is, by injection). The hot debate at the moment is whether to give one big dose of three drugs intravenously so that symptoms appear all at once, or to give smaller doses by mouth over a longer period of time, so that the patient gets cumulatively sicker. You get better more quickly after one big dose and this is the preferred treatment when using chemotherapy to treat curable cancers. This is because the long-term use of lower doses, as with radiotherapy, has a risk of causing other types of cancer to develop as a delayed effect of treatment.

Chemotherapy affects all cells, but especially those of the skin, gut and bone marrow, which are cells that divide the fastest, and this accounts for the main side effects of hair loss, nausea and a lowered blood count. You can be given drugs for nausea, but if nausea is expected to be severe, a patient may be admitted to hospital for her chemo – although this is rarely necessary. Some drugs can cause mouth ulcers, while other drugs have no side effects at all. Chemo affects people in different ways – some patients only become more tired as a result of it. Get as much rest during treatment as you can, and 'up' your protein intake to help your body withstand any side effects. If you don't feel like eating, substitute high-protein drinks at meal times.

Because chemo affects the ability of bone marrow to produce platelets, which in turn affects the clotting of the blood, avoid cutting or injuring yourself during treatment, and use an electric razor. Your white blood cell count may be lowered as well, so avoid crowds or exposure to cold germs, as it will be harder for you to fight off an infection. Also, tell your doctor if you experience any of the following symptoms as a result of chemo: sweating; chills; sore throat; frequent, persistent sores; vaginal itching; oozing gums; bruising or long, heavy periods.

Chemotherapy treatment

Treatment takes place over anything from one to fourteen days, then there is a rest period for a few weeks. The length of chemo treatment depends on the type of cancer and how well it responds to drugs. Prolonged use of chemo can make difficult the finding of veins in the arm for intravenous treatment. Each drug is active only against certain types of cancer – that is, it will kill some of that cancer in some patients. Chemo has been very effective in treating childhood leukaemia and Hodgkin's disease, as well as some other rare cancers such as cancer of the testicles and ovarian germ-cell tumours (that is, tumours arising from any of the embryonic cells that have the potential to develop into eggs). Compared to radiotherapy, the acute side effects of chemotherapy are more drastic, but the delayed late effects are less distressing, although in some situations, second cancers may occur – and to keep this to a minimum, doctors try to use as few as possible of the drugs which belong to a group called 'alkylating agents'. This group includes cyclophosphamide, mustine, chlorambucil and melphalan.

Adjuvant chemotherapy

Adjuvant chemotherapy (see pp. 141 – 142) is given if your cancer has an inclination to relapse, as with breast cancer. It is given at a time when there are no other symptoms of the disease but because doctors believe that the cancer could still reappear. But if the chance of recurrence is not high for your particular cancer, it is not usually advisable to opt for extra chemo; if you do, keep the treatment as short as possible. This is because, apart from side effects, chemo can interfere with your ovaries: if you are pre-menopausal your periods may become more erratic or could stop altogether; or you may get other menopausal symptoms – or you could even become infertile.

But your menopausal symptoms could disappear, and your periods return to normal, *after* chemo: the younger you are, and the shorter the treatment, the more likely your ovaries are to recover.

Sometimes the use of chemo and radiotherapy together can cause new cancers like acute leukaemia to arise, especially if you have a primary cancer of the ovary and have been taking chlorambucil or other oral drugs for long periods of time.

Chemotherapy and pregnancy

A pregnancy conceived during chemotherapy has a higher-than-normal risk of miscarriage and birth defects. What the risk factors would be if a pregnancy is started *after* chemotherapy treatment has been completed is not yet known.

Side effects of chemotherapy

Side effects include nausea and vomiting, loss of appetite, fatigue and diarrhoea. However, chemotherapy affects people in different ways, and many patients have few or none of these symptoms, and only feel more tired when taking chemotherapy.

Some people lose their hair with chemotherapy, but this is not always the case. Hair loss usually results when drugs are combined together: for instance, whenever Adriamycin is used hair loss may occur. Carboplatin and a drug called ifosfamide do not cause hair loss. But even if just a single drug is used, if you are on and off chemo for twelve months some hair loss is inevitable. If a woman is susceptible to hair loss, it will occur within the first two to three months of starting chemo. Although all hair may be lost in some susceptible women, no one ever goes bald *permanently* – hair regrows when chemo is finished, and sometimes in better condition than before. Curly hair can sometimes grow back straight, and some hair can regrow a different colour. If your hair starts to fall out during treatment, wear a hairnet to bed at night and under a wig during the daytime – this way, the hair loss is less traumatic and no one need know about it. Opt for a synthetic wig, which is lighter than a natural one and can be looked after more easily at home.

HORMONE THERAPY

If a cancer arises in a hormone-sensitive organ such as the womb or breast, the cancer may be stimulated into further growth by hormonal messages – particularly from the hormone oestrogen which is produced naturally in the body of a woman of child-bearing age and which fluctuates during the menstrual cycle. A patient with this type of cancer can be treated with an artificial 'inhibiting' hormone, which 'tells' the cells to stop dividing. (The other options are surgery or radiation to the ovary.) Tamoxifen, for example, is an anti-oestrogen which can produce a remission in breast cancer in women and men of any age, and it is also useful in uterine cancer. There are no unpleasant side effects. The dose needed depends on how much oestrogen there is to be neutralised: menstruating women need higher doses. Hormone therapy was first used in 1902.

OTHER ORTHODOX TREATMENTS

An additional group of drugs sometimes used to treat cancer patients are known as 'biological response modifiers' or 'immuno-stimulants' (see also p.211). An immuno-stimulant is a substance which, when injected into a cancer patient, helps to stimulate her immune system to fight the cancer. This approach, called immunotherapy, should not be confused with immunology, which is the study of immunity and everything connected with the defence mechanisms of the body. Many scientifically minded complementary therapists also use it, as you will read later.

Most orthodox doctors do not think very highly of this approach, believing that any resulting effects are too weak to be of practical use. There have been at least three periods of enthusiasm for immunotherapy: in the early 1900s, in 1960 – 75 and in 1987 – 9. Three substances in particular that you may have heard of in connection with this type of treatment are:

Interferon – this is a substance produced by the body in response to a virus, which stops the virus from multiplying. It works by preventing viruses from harnessing the cells' normal dividing mechanisms to reproduce themselves. Synthetically produced interferon has been used to normalise 'hair-cell' leukaemia in 90 per cent of cases and has shrunk 15 per cent of skin and kidney cancers.

Studies with interferon's effectiveness against each kind of cancer are still continuing – it has already taken twelve years to get this far. Trials incorporating interferon with other conventional treatments such as surgery or radiotherapy have only just begun, and will take another five to ten years to complete. Interferon is not quite the miracle cure that the press made it out to be in 1977: it is on the toxic side, and is certainly not as effective as most cytotoxic drugs.

Interleukin 2 – this is a hormone that drives T-lymphocytes, a type of white blood cell: it puts more of these lymphocytes into the circulation and in the area of the cancer. It is now three years since interleukin 2 was made available in unlimited amounts for clinical trials, and so far improvement has been seen only in skin and kidney cancers, but less than half the main types of cancer have been formally tested with this substance to date.

And there are still problems with the dosage: only extremely high doses have been tested, and work is still in progress to define the optimum dose, as well as to find out whether this drug can be incorporated into more conventional treatments for cancer. Reactions in patients range from flu-like symptoms to a coma, with the latter category requiring admission to an intensive-care unit. It is too early to pass final judgement on this drug, although it does offer some hope to patients with tumour spread who haven't responded to more conventional treatment.

Interleukin 3 – this substance, despite its name, is not related to interleukin 2; it acts by regulating types of blood cells called 'polymorphs', scavengers which clean the bloodstream by eating cancer cells. It is sometimes given to patients on chemotherapy, as it gives their blood twice the usual level of polymorphs, which helps prevent infection and allows higher doses of chemo to be given. Interleukin 3 has its drawbacks as well – it can waterlog the tissues – and research on it continues.

MONOCLONAL ANTIBODIES

One of the newest diagnostic techniques for cancer is monoclonal antibodies, which are antibodies produced artificially in a laboratory from mice cells, and which react against various types of cancer. They are used to detect cancer in the human body via the bloodstream, and can help determine the extent of a tumour. They can also help to make predictions about how a patient will respond to treatment. Monoclonal antibodies work by recognising and sticking to cancer cells and so are used as the carrier for a radio-isotope or anti-cancer drug. They are currently being tested as a method to check whether cancer has spread to the lymph glands under the arm. This way, surgery to remove a lymph gland to check for cancer spread will become unnecessary.

There has been considerable discussion about the possibility of using monoclonal antibodies attached to high doses of drugs or radioactive isotopes and targeted at the tumour to help kill it. This is known as a 'magic bullet'. There are still some problems with magic bullets, however: first, the bullets must be able to distinguish more completely between normal cells and cancer cells; second, bullets don't always stick tightly enough; and third, most monoclonal antibodies are of mouse origin, and this creates antibodies in the body against the mouse cells, instead of stimulating the immune system to create antibodies against the *cancer*. *If* these problems can be ironed out, armed monoclonal antibodies, or 'magic bullets', will be a stronger weapon among orthodox medicine's arsenal of cancer treatments.

NUCLEAR MAGNETIC RESONANCE

A patient may find that she is being scanned with the help of the latest development in nuclear medicine: a nuclear magnetic resonance (NMR) machine. This is where the patient is placed in a magnetic field and radio pulses are emitted which stimulate signals in the atoms of the body. Cancer cells emit radio-frequency signals which differ from those of healthy cells, which can be picked up and displayed on a monitor screen. At present many doctors believe that NMR's prohibitive cost outweighs any small advantage it might have over the CAT scan, in which 'slices' of the body are recorded with an X-ray scanner (see p.51 for a more detailed description of a CAT scan). The only outstanding advantage of NMR at the moment is when scanning the brain for a tumour.

A CRITIQUE OF ORTHODOX MEDICINE

Orthodox medicine has often been accused of focusing on the disease rather than on the person manifesting the disease. This stems from the Cartesian philosophy developed by the eighteenth-century Frenchman René Descartes, which has had a strong influence on Western medicine. It states that the human body is ruled by mechanical laws and that it is separate from the immortal soul. In other words, 'The whole is the sum of its parts.'

This approach to the patient, however, is slowly being replaced with a more 'whole' or 'holistic' view of a patient. According to John Shepherd, a gynaecological oncologist at the Royal Marsden Hospital, London, the Cartesian view used to be the specialist approach, but a 'good' doctor will treat both patient *and* symptoms. Michael Baum, Professor of Surgery at

King's College Hospital, London, adds, 'I have no doubt at all that any good doctor, trained within any of our medical schools, should approach his or her work with patients in a holistic manner.'

Many specialists realise that other treatments, besides merely physical ones, are of great value. John Shepherd feels that counselling is very important – he believes that a doctor should ideally become involved in the patient's problem. And although orthodox doctors have had a reputation in the past for not looking at complementary treatments, Shepherd believes that this is changing and that doctors just don't have all the answers.

A few medical schools, along with the Royal College of Nursing, are including basic acupuncture and holistic health care on their agendas. Orthopaedic surgeons are now recommending osteopathy. Some patient support groups at cancer hospitals are now offering to teach meditation and self-hypnosis for pain. Psychotherapy is often available, with patient care continuing even after the patient's discharge from hospital, for as long as the patient needs it.

The British Holistic Medical Association (see the list of addresses, p.283), formed in 1983 for doctors and other health-care workers, aims to bring together both orthodox and complementary medicine. (For more on the bridge between orthodox and complementary medicine, see pp.172 – 173.)

5

Ovarian Cancer

The ovaries are two, small, egg-producing glands the size of olives, located on either side of the uterus. Every month one of the ovaries produces an egg which passes down the Fallopian tube into the uterus. If the egg is not fertilised, it passes out of the uterus along with the uterine lining as part of the monthly period. The ovaries also produce the female sex hormones, oestrogen and progesterone. As a woman gets older, less and less of these hormones are made, egg production winds down and her periods become more irregular and finally stop. This brings on the menopause, usually between the ages of forty-eight and fifty-two.

THE FACTS

- **UK incidence.** In 1984, 5,160 new cases were registered in the UK (4 per cent of all cancers).
- **England and Wales five-year survival rate.** From 1981, 28 per cent of cases were alive five years later.
- **UK mortality.** In 1986, 4,345 patients died (6 per cent of all cancer deaths).

Approximately 5,000 women in the UK contract ovarian cancer every year. In 75 per cent of cases it has spread beyond the ovaries before it is diagnosed. Most women who get this cancer are over forty-five, but about 1,000 women annually under the age of forty also get it. About 4,000 women die from the disease every year – that's twice as many as die from cervical cancer. In fact, ovarian cancer is the commonest gynaecological malignancy, accounting for 54 per cent of the deaths resulting from a malignant growth which originates in a woman's reproductive organs.

Worldwide, generally only 25 per cent of women survive five years, and this statistic has remained largely unchanged over the last twenty to thirty years. However, more women with an *advanced* ovarian cancer are surviving at least two to three years. It must be remembered that these statistics are very general, and that every case of cancer is different, with individual patients often beating the general medical odds. The highest ovarian cancer incidence rate (the number of people contracting it) is in Scandinavia, the lowest in Japan. The chicken is the only other animal that dies from ovarian cancer – that is because it is a super-ovulator. This means that chickens ovulate all the time, as compared to human females who ovulate monthly – thus a chicken's risk of ovarian cancer is greater than a woman's, as the disease is directly related to the length of time that the ovaries are active. And, yes, battery hens get more ovarian cancer than free-range hens!

SYMPTOMS

According to David Oram, consultant gynaecological surgeon at the London Hospital, 'The problem with ovarian cancer is that there are no real symptoms, no pre-invasive state, no high-risk population, no early screening test. It is also in an inaccessible organ.' The symptoms are, indeed, vague: abdominal pain and/or swelling; gastro-intestinal problems such as indigestion, nausea, persistent constipation, diarrhoea, a bloated feeling; weight loss; urinary or pelvic pressure; backache; occasional shortness of breath; ankle swelling; and, rarely, abnormal bleeding. A few women have felt a mass, but a very small percentage have had no symptoms at all.

Up to 90 per cent of ovarian cancers are thought to develop from epithelial or 'surface' lining cells of the ovary, while the majority of the remaining 10 per cent develop from a germ cell which is the stage before development of an egg cell. These tumours are called 'germ-cell' tumours: they are aggressive tumours in terms of speed of growth and only affect younger women, during the period of greatest sex hormone activity between the ages of fifteen and twenty-five. The germ cell is the same kind of cell as that involved in the development of a foetus. Most germ-cell tumours, if caught in time, can be cured by chemotherapy.

RISK FACTORS

No one knows what causes ovarian cancer, although it is more common among women who have had no children. By studying women who contracted the cancer, however, cancer specialists have worked backwards to a set of 'risk' factors. These include: having no children or having your first child after the age of twenty-five (both risk factors relate to the fact that the ovaries have been active – ovulating monthly – without the 'rest period' that a pregnancy gives to the ovaries); using talcum powder around the vaginal area, as particles of powder can travel up into the female organs and lodge there; excess coffee drinking; the mumps virus; an adolescent rubella infection; and the use of non-contraceptive oestrogens (ie HRT; this is because some ovarian cancers have oestrogen receptors on them). Age itself is a risk factor, with women most vulnerable over the age of fifty. It also appears to be a disease more associated with the middle and upper classes, so there are social and economic factors involved, but doctors do not yet know which ones.

The family link

While many of these risk factors are theoretical, the strongest one appears to be family link. If your mother or sister had ovarian cancer, your chance of getting it is increased. The risk is even higher when two or more close female relatives have had the disease.

Certain families do seem to be prone to groups of cancers – ovarian, breast and bowel cancers form one such group – which can affect different generations of the same family. At the Royal Marsden Hospital in London, ovarian cancer patients are asked about other female members of their family, and if they are considered to be at risk, they are offered an annual consultation, pelvic examination, CA 125 blood test (see p.50) and screening with ultrasound. The heredity factor is considered similar to that of breast cancer.

If you move from a country where the risk is low to a country where the risk is high, your children and your children's children will take on the same risk as the women of the high-risk country. This happened when Japanese women left Japan, a low-risk country for ovarian disease, and settled in the United States, a high-risk country. Why this happens is not known, but it does point the finger at environmental and dietary factors.

Risk factors, though, must be kept in perspective – having one or even many risk factors does not mean that you will contract ovarian cancer. As no one knows what causes it, this only means that you are *statistically* more likely to contract ovarian cancer.

DIAGNOSTIC TESTS

If ovarian cancer is suspected, your GP and your hospital doctor will do a series of tests. The first thing your GP might do is to give you a bi-manual pelvic examination, in which he/she feels the lower abdomen and then the internal organs of the pelvis via the vagina and rectum. In this way a doctor might find a mass that began in an ovary, Fallopian tube or the uterus. (It is a good idea for every woman to have a bi-manual pelvic examination annually – see 'Screening for Ovarian Cancer', p.64.)

Your doctor will then refer you to hospital for further tests. These tests can include:

1 *Ultrasound scan.* This procedure, similar to the one used to screen pregnant women, can spot an enlargement or an abnormality of the ovaries which may indicate a cyst or tumour, and even measure the size of it. Sound waves are used to make up a picture of the inside of the abdomen, liver and pelvis, which is then shown on a computer screen. About 1

litre (2 pints) of water must be drunk beforehand, as a full
bladder displaces the intestines upwards to allow a clearer
picture of the pelvis, uterus and ovaries.

2 *Computer-assisted tomography (CAT) scan.* This is a type of X-
ray which can show the size and position of a cancer. On the
day of the scan you will be asked not to eat or drink for four
hours before your appointment. Two hours before your scan,
and again in the X-ray department, you will drink special
liquid that shows up on an X-ray. Just before the scan a
similar liquid is put into your back passage and a tampon put
in your vagina: this ensures a clear picture. The machine
then takes a number of photographs and feeds them into a
computer, to compile a detailed look at the inside of the
abdomen, liver and pelvis. The whole procedure can take up
to three hours, with several waiting periods, so bring a friend
for company.

3 *Barium enema.* This is a special X-ray of the bowel. The bowel
must be empty for a clear picture, and so a laxative is taken
the day before and nothing is eaten or drunk before the
morning test. During the test a mixture of barium and air is
passed into the back passage and held in the bowel until all
the X-rays can be seen. A doctor watches the passage of the
barium through the bowel on an X-ray screen, checking for
abnormalities. There may be white stools and some
constipation for a few days after treatment, but this is
normal.

4 *Intravenous urogram (IVU or IVP).* Sometimes the spread of
cancer can interfere with the kidneys, ureters (tubes con-
necting the kidneys and bladder), urethra (tube passing urine
from the bladder to the exterior) or bladder, and this test will
show up any abnormalities in the urinary system. A dye is
injected into a vein which then travels to the kidneys. A
doctor watching this on an X-ray screen can spot any
abnormalities. Some people feel hot and flushed for a few
minutes immediately after injection with the dye, but if you
have any allergic tendencies, mention them to the staff, as
they can inject you with something different which causes no
reaction at all. The test takes an hour.

5 *Lymphangiogram (or lymphogram).* This is a slightly more
complicated X-ray involving a dye. In many hospitals it has
been replaced by the CAT scan. It checks for any

abnormalities of the lymph nodes in the abdomen and pelvis. A blue dye is injected into the upper part of each foot close to the toes, which passes through the lymphatic vessels to the lymph nodes in the abdomen and pelvis – the blue dye shows up on the X-ray.

After this, a tiny cut is made on each foot after a local anaesthetic is applied, and an oily substance is gradually injected which also shows up on the X-ray. The doctor watches the progress of these two substances on the X-ray, looking for abnormalities. The test takes two to three hours. A stitch is then put in each cut, which is taken out a week later. For the next forty-eight hours the skin can appear greenish and the urine a blue-green colour while the dye is being excreted, but this is only a temporary effect.

6 *Abdominal fluid aspiration.* This is performed if there has been a build-up of fluid in the abdomen. After a local anaesthetic numbs the area, a syringe draws off a sample of the fluid, which is then checked under a microscope for cancer cells.

7 *Laparoscopy.* This small operation (see p.55 for a description) allows doctors to look at the ovaries and the surrounding area with a laparoscope (a sort of mini-telescope) and to take a small tissue sample for microscopic examination. It can also be used before major surgery if a mass is suspected but cannot be seen on a scan. A few stitches close the cut. Afterwards there may be a few days of uncomfortable wind, as this procedure disturbs the bowel temporarily.

STAGING OVARIAN CANCER

The 'staging' of a cancer is determining the degree of spread. About 5 per cent of ovarian tumours are not primary ovarian carcinomas at all, but tumours that have spread from their origin in the breast or gastro-intestinal tract. Ovarian cancer is staged as follows:

Stage 1

Growth limited to one or both ovaries; around 75 – 90 per cent of patients survive five years (this is a 'median' survival rate).

Stage 2

Growth involving the ovaries and lower abdomen. This stage represents only 10 – 15 per cent of cases; on average, 50 per cent of patients have a five-year survival.

Stage 3

Cancer has spread to the rest of the abdominal organs except the liver, and there is possible lymph node involvement. On average, up to 15 per cent of patients have a five-year survival. Unfortunately, this advanced stage includes the majority of patients with ovarian cancer.

Stage 4

Growth involving the ovaries with distant metastases, or spread to the liver. On average, less than 5 per cent of patients survive five years.

GRADING OVARIAN CANCER

The 'grade' of a cancer is a measure of how aggressive it is – and this can be discovered by looking at the cells under a microscope and giving them a grade 1, 2 or 3. Well-differentiated tumours are those which look the most like normal tissue and tend to spread more slowly (grade 1); moderately well-differentiated tumours are less like normal tissue in their cell construction and spread more quickly (grade 2); and poorly differentiated tumours are furthest from normal tissue and tend to spread quickly (grade 3). Obviously the grade of a tumour can make a patient's prospects better or worse at any 'stage' of the cancer.

TREATMENT

The treatment of ovarian cancer is tied in with its stages.

Stage 1

For Stage 1 the cure rate with *surgery* is high (see p.55). This involves removing both ovaries, even when only one is affected, and usually the uterus and Fallopian tubes as well, although for a woman with only one ovary affected who wishes to save her fertility, it may be possible to remove one ovary only and allow the woman time to try for a family. This option must be discussed carefully with her doctor, as there is a chance of relapse.

The reason so much is taken away at this early stage is that there is usually a high incidence of microscopic disease in the uterus and remaining good ovary, and both are common sites for recurrence. For a stage 1 ovarian cancer, grades 1 and 2 have an 80 per cent chance or more of a cure; grades 3 and 4 slightly less, and may need some additional treatment after surgery.

Stage 2

As much of the tumour as possible is removed by *surgery* (see p.55) – this means both ovaries, the uterus and Fallopian tubes, and at this point fertility cannot be saved. If there is minimal tumour left after surgery (it may not be possible to remove all the tumour if, for example, it is clinging to a vital organ), some centres use radiotherapy to reduce the risk of the disease recurring. If a large mass of the tumour has to be left behind, radiotherapy is less useful and *chemotherapy* is given.

Stages 3 and 4

Surgery is still the main approach at this stage (see p.55). Even when the cancer is widely spread, it is sometimes possible to remove all or nearly all of the visible cancer – this is because the tumour does not always invade tissues deeply. The large fatty sheet, or omentum, which overlies the abdomen is removed too.

A sample of the lymph nodes may also be taken to check the degree of spread. Patients whose largest tumour mass left behind after surgery is less than 2 cm (0.75 inch) diameter will respond better to treatment and have a higher survival rate.

SURGERY

As we have seen, some kind of surgery is always the first treatment for ovarian cancer (see p.35 for a general introduction to surgery). The need for good surgery at any stage of ovarian cancer is all-important – 'good' in the sense that it is performed by an experienced surgeon who has the time to look carefully for spread and to remove all the cancer that he sees. Whatever 'stage' the surgeon deems the cancer to be at will determine the treatment a woman receives – stage is more important than the size of a tumour as a prognostic indicator (that is, in showing the likely course and outcome of the cancer), according to Dr Ian Jacobs at the London Hospital.

If, for example, a tumour were diagnosed as stage 1 when it was really stage 3, no chemotherapy would be given, as stage 1 tumours are not treated with chemotherapy. This could ultimately affect survival. The survival rate in the UK for ovarian cancer is worse than in Scandinavia and slightly worse than that in the USA – and some specialists believe that this could be the result of improper staging. This might also explain the high recurrence of ovarian cancer and why up to 50 per cent of patients with apparently localised disease die.

It is not always possible to detect a subclinical tumour (that is, a tumour which is suspected, but which is not sufficiently developed to produce definite signs and symptoms in the patient), but an experienced ovarian surgeon will know what to look for. Says Jacobs, 'Perfect surgery on every patient would actually improve survival rates slightly.' In fact careful surgery will ensure that 90 per cent of those with stage 1 disease get past the critical five-year period.

So what is a woman to do? First, ensure that her GP or gynaecologist refers her to an experienced ovarian cancer surgeon.

Decisions about surgery

A woman may be faced with some decisions regarding her ovarian surgery. For instance, if during the small operation called a laparoscopy, where the surgeon makes a small cut in the lower abdomen and inserts a laparoscope to look at the ovaries and take a small tissue sample for microscopic examination (see p.52), it is decided that the biopsy is malignant, the surgeon may want to carry on into a full operation, or laparotomy, to remove the tumour. You, however, may want a second opinion on this.

Also, some surgeons may want to do what is called a 'second-look' laparotomy, a second major operation some months after the first, in order to see if any tumour is still present and to give a second shot at tumour removal. Discuss this option carefully, or get a second opinion, because recent trials have shown that there is no benefit to be derived from a 'second look'. The use of a 'second-look' laparotomy is now largely restricted to research.

Unfortunately, when ovarian cancer spreads, it tends to skip stage 2 and involves the whole abdomen, so it would be unwise to pin all your hopes on surgery. Surgery cannot always extend life, but it may improve the quality of it, and those who have lots of disease left after surgery do have a poorer prognosis (forecast of the course of disease). Advanced surgical techniques have made extensive surgery possible even for the old and infirm, so the rule seems to be to have as much tumour removed as possible.

Prophylactic oophorectomy

Prophylactic oophorectomy is the surgical removal of the ovaries as a preventative measure – it could be considered by high-risk women (those with a family history, those over forty-five) during any kind of pelvic surgery after completing their families. Up to 20 per cent of ovarian cancers might be prevented by this method. But there is no need to fear that a surgeon would be overkeen to whip out your ovaries even if you were 'high-risk', especially if you are a younger woman. A survey conducted by David Oram of UK surgeons who regularly perform hysterectomies revealed that less than 1 per cent would remove ovaries in women in the thirty-five to thirty-nine age group, only 2.4 per cent in the forty to forty-four age group, and only 20.4 per cent would remove them in the forty-five to forty-nine age group. This is because no surgeon likes to remove healthy tissue, and it may be that the ovaries serve functions which we haven't discovered yet.

Also, prophylactic oophorectomy is not guaranteed to work: some women at very high risk may get cancer in the same area as their ovaries even twenty years after the preventative operation. This is a very rare occurrence, but it happened to four out of twenty-five women in a study conducted in Los Angeles, and the reason is that an inherited tendency towards malignancy can be present in the general tissue of the abdomen, and not just confined to the ovaries.

Another reason to consider this procedure carefully is that it is necessary to take one hundred ovaries out in order to stop one cancer developing, a lot of unnecessary surgery for the other ninety-nine women.

Peritoneoscopy

In the USA, and sometimes in the UK, a procedure called peritoneoscopy is used to see if there is any residual disease left after surgery. Under a local anaesthetic a blunt needle is inserted in the abdomen below the navel. Air or carbon dioxide is pumped into the abdomen which lifts up the abdomen wall and allows a tiny microscope to view the liver and undersurfaces of the abdomen.

Minute tumour nodules can be detected and biopsied (that is, samples can be removed for examination), and any excess fluid can be sampled for malignant cells. The National Cancer Institute in the USA revealed in one study using peritoneoscopy that 56 per cent of patients who were thought to be stage 2 – that is, with their disease limited to the pelvis – were actually stage 3. These patients would have received no treatment for disease in the upper abdomen!

RADIOTHERAPY

As an alternative to surgical removal, ovaries can be irradiated to put them out of action.

Radiotherapy (see p.36 for a general introduction) can also be used after surgery when there is only a little tumour left; otherwise chemotherapy is used. Radiotherapy should not be used when there is a lot of post-surgery tumour left, as this means irradiating the whole abdomen which produces too many side effects, some of which could be permanent.

The principle of radiotherapy is to use as high a dose as possible on the tumour without causing damage to the normal tissues. Cancer cells are destroyed by the radiation damaging their genetic material, making them unable to divide.

The value of post-operative radiotherapy for ovarian cancer is debatable: it's more worthwhile if the growth has spread outside the ovary, but because the abdomen has such a low tolerance of radiotherapy, some oncologists don't like using it at all. The normal side effects of radiotherapy include nausea and vomiting, loss of appetite, fatigue and diarrhoea.

Complications arise from the following factors: the total dose, the volume of tissue treated, the patient's age and any previous history of inflammatory bowel disease or adhesions from prior surgery. These all increase the risk of radiation-induced toxicity (poisoning). Irreversible damage to the small intestine can occur as a result of high doses of radiation (e.g. from about 4,500 – 5,000 rads), and it is always wise to discuss any long-term implications of high doses of radiation of the lower abdomen with your radiographer and doctor. Radiotherapy is a more apt therapy for cancers of the cervix and uterus, which tend to be more localised.

CHEMOTHERAPY

Chemotherapy (see p.39 for a general introduction) can cure 90 per cent of patients with germ-cell tumours, and between one in ten and one in twenty patients with non-germ cell (epithelial) tumours. In addition, in the latter groups it can cause major shrinkage of tumours in up to half the patients, making them comfortable for between six and eighteen months on average. Those that do best on chemotherapy have very little cancer left. Treatment duration varies, depending on the amount of tumour, from as little as two months up to one or two years. Chemo can make the spaces between relapses as long as possible, giving a patient with advanced disease a few more years of active, comfortable life.

Combinations of more than one cytotoxic drug seem more effective in reducing a tumour's size than a single drug. Chemo-therapy tends to be given every three to four weeks for six or more cycles of treatment, although it isn't yet clear whether long-term remissions or cures will result from this approach. If there is no response after several treatments, the drugs should be changed.

A recent innovation in giving chemotherapy to ovarian cancer patients is injection of the drugs through the abdominal wall, which is good in principle as it reaches the site of the cancer directly, but as yet there is no proof that it works any better than the conventional injection into an arm vein. Kidney function is always checked before starting chemo, as this organ is important for the elimination of cytotoxic drugs quickly from the body. One other approach being tried in specialist units is to give five to ten times the normal dose of the drug, after having taken 300 ml (½ pint) of bone marrow from the patient. The bone marrow is stored in a special refrigerator, and given back to the patient when she develops a suppression of her blood count from the drugs. This is done because chemotherapy affects the bone marrow's ability to produce platelets, and so the damaged bone marrow can be replaced by the patient's own.

Bone marrow is taken when carboplatin is used, one of the newer platinum-derived cytotoxic drugs, as it can reduce the number of red blood cells in the bloodstream. A hearing test may also be given before and after treatment, when receiving cisplatin (see below) as this drug can affect your hearing, but this is not a problem with the newer carboplatin.

Though ovarian cancer is considered to be more 'chemo-sensitive' than cervical or uterine cancer, some doctors question whether it is necessary to use chemotherapy treatment for every patient with this type of cancer. Again, discuss your options carefully about chemotherapy: whether, for instance, to try a single drug orally which is moderately effective with few side effects, or to try a combination of drugs given intravenously which is better for reducing the tumour size and allowing a longer remission, but which has more side effects. And although you may get better more quickly on the intravenous chemo, there is no evidence that it is any better for a cure in the long term.

Side effects of chemotherapy are discussed on p.41.

Cisplatin and carboplatin

One drug used frequently in chemotherapy to treat ovarian cancer is cisplatin, another platinum-derived compound which came before carboplatin. Although both are equally effective, carboplatin produçes less nausea in a patient.

All cytotoxic drugs can make you cumulatively sicker over a series of treatments, but carboplatin makes you cumulatively *less* sick. This is because this version of platinum is less toxic at high doses. It is also a more expensive drug, and at present more difficult to obtain, in part because it has not been fully evaluated in all stages of the disease. Still, if severe nausea is putting you off finishing your course of chemotherapy, it is worth asking whether you can be treated with carboplatin. At the time of writing the Royal Marsden Hospital in London is testing high doses of carboplatin on the early stages of ovarian cancer with excellent results.

Case Study – OVARIAN CANCER

Barbara Manning had a history of ovarian cysts and at the age of thirty-five had an operation to remove two benign cysts. Three years later she returned to her GP with the same symptoms: slight pain in lower abdomen and down one leg, and a vaginal discharge which became bloodstained after sexual intercourse. Her GP sent her to a gynaecologist who believed the cause to be more cysts, but advised a total hysterectomy as a preventative measure, which would also remove her ovaries (one quarter of an ovary had been removed in the previous operation). Barbara agreed, as she had 'finished' her family.

When she came round after surgery she felt 'dreadful' and 'ill at ease'. Her gynaecologist told her that she'd had two malignant growths – one on each ovary – and the right-sided growth had been adhering to the bowel. The gynaecologist had scraped the bowel very well and was confident that he had got it all but he recommended a course of radiotherapy to make sure.

She found her radiotherapy treatment 'very traumatic'. It consisted of five days a week for six weeks, during which her bowels reacted badly. She had constant diarrhoea and a feeling of nausea, and the medication she was offered could help only the nausea. She was allowed no baths or fruit and vegetables during the five-day treatment sessions. She lost all her body hair (but not the hair on her head), which didn't grow back properly. Her weight dropped from 50 to 41 kg (8 to 6½ stone), and she needed a week off in the middle of treatment because her skin was badly burnt.

After radiotherapy treatment Barbara felt weak, but still went off on a holiday. Five days into her holiday, however, her right side swelled up painfully and so she flew back home. Her doctors decided to try 'drug therapy' (this was in pre-chemotherapy days), which consisted of two pills taken together twice a week, followed by a blood test to ensure that her white corpuscles were not being unduly affected. The treatment lasted eighteen months, during which Barbara felt very unwell and put on weight: she reach 63 kg (10 stone). Gradually, however, she began to feel better; the swelling began to subside after six months, and at the end of eighteen months had completely gone. As soon as she came off the drugs she lost the excess weight, and so wonders if there were steroids in the pills. Her only remaining symptoms were bowel trouble, either severe diarrhoea or constipation, probably a carry-over from her radiotherapy treatment.

The specialist decided to operate again, to have a look. No cancer could be seen. Barbara was now forty. Afterwards she had some health problems which she attributes to the actual cancer (piles, spastic colon, kidney stones and a gall bladder which needed removing), but, fourteen years later she is still cancer-free. She had six-monthly check-ups for five years, and now has them annually.

Although her bowel still gives her problems, Barbara eats what she likes, but avoids bran and cereals. Despite the lingering side effects of some of her treatments, Barbara feels grateful to be alive and basically well sixteen years after a diagnosis of ovarian cancer.

HORMONES

A woman's hormones seem to be linked in some way to ovarian cancer: like breast cancer, it is a hormone-receptive cancer. In the ongoing study on the island of Guernsey, it has been shown that some women have abnormal amounts of certain hormones in their urine years before they contract not only breast cancer, but ovarian cancer as well. However, these abnormal hormone levels are not strong enough markers to tell doctors in advance who will develop breast/ovarian cancer and who will not: only 5 – 10 per cent of these women develop cancer. Unfortunately, urinary hormone levels don't narrow the field enough to warrant using them as a screening test. If you have breast cancer, you have a higher risk of contracting ovarian cancer, and vice versa. In fact, the hormone drug tamoxifen, which is used in the treatment of breast cancer, has been shown in some studies to help ovarian cancer.

The hormonal link is most striking when you realise that the majority of women who get ovarian cancer develop it around the menopause: the peak incidence is between the ages of fifty-five and fifty-nine. Ovarian cancer patients usually have a history of hormonal imbalance and misfunction, and if the hormone link can be proved, it may turn out that ovarian cancer is actually started by the pituitary gland (the endocrine gland at the base of the brain; it controls many of the other endocrine glands).

HORMONE REPLACEMENT THERAPY

Whether the ovaries are irradiated or surgically removed, the result is the loss of oestrogen and a premature menopause. Symptoms include vaginal dryness, dry skin, a decrease in sexual desire and hot and cold flushes, although not every woman suffers all, or necessarily any, symptoms. Protection against osteoporosis (weakening of the bones) and atherosclerosis (narrowing of the blood vessels) is also lost.

That is why, provided that there is no indication that her tumour was/is hormone-dependent, it is important for women with missing or inactivated ovaries to have hormone replacement therapy (HRT), which prevents or reverses menopausal symptoms and helps guard against osteoporosis. However, as the data about the hormone dependence of ovarian cancer is still unresolved it is advised that HRT is not started until after the first year after surgery (other medication will be given in the meantime). When used, HRT is given as an oestrogen-progesterone combination, as oestrogen given by itself is associated with an increased risk of endometrial cancer, and this would be particularly relevant to an ovarian cancer patient who has retained her uterus.

THE CONTRACEPTIVE PILL

Although there is no evidence to suggest that HRT protects or endangers with regard to ovarian cancer, there is strong evidence that the contraceptive pill *protects* against this cancer. The degree of protection is directly proportional to the degree of usage. Explains David Oram, 'Ovarian cancer is rarely found among women who took the pill for ten years; it is uncommonly found among women who took it for six years; it is infrequently found among those who took it for two years; and it then starts occurring among women who took it for six months or not at all.' Having said this, it still looks as though six months on the contraceptive pill offers some protection. Studies do not go back further than ten years of pill use. The risk, globally, is reduced to 50 per cent of that of a non-pill user, and in some cases, to as low as 20 per cent (according to Professor Martin Vessey), when the pill has been taken for ten years.

From studies, it appears that women who took the pill between the ages of twenty-five and thirty-five have less ovarian cancer in their fifties and sixties. What isn't clear, however, is whether this protection is lifelong or diminishes slowly over a period of years – it *is* thought that pill users whose mothers died of ovarian cancer or have some other family link with the disease would have less protection from the pill than other women. But again, how much decrease in protection isn't yet clear.

The pill 'protects' by mimicking pregnancy, which 'rests' the ovaries. This means that the ovaries are not having to produce a monthly egg – think of chickens, who are more likely to die of ovarian cancer because of all the eggs they produce (see page 48)! There may be a negative side to the pill, though: the possibility of cardiovascular complications and the hotly disputed but possible link to breast cancer.

However, as oncologist Tim Oliver puts it, 'Because the research around the pill and breast cancer is so contradictory, the actual risk must be very low, whereas the protection provided by the pill against ovarian cancer is so clear-cut that it must be worth taking the pill for that reason alone.'

BI-MANUAL PELVIC EXAMINATION

There is some controversy over whether women over the age of forty-five, and high-risk women, should be given a bi-manual pelvic examination (see p.50) every year by their doctor as a preventative measure against ovarian cancer. David Oram claims that it takes 10,000 examinations to pick up one unsuspected case of the disease. This is because the entire abdominal cavity is capable of expanding to accommodate a growing mass, so a tumour may not be felt until it is the size of a small grapefruit.

However, in a post-menopausal woman the ovaries shrink to an average size of 2 cm (0.75 inch), so if the doctor can feel the ovaries in a post-menopausal woman, something is wrong. In a *pre*-menopausal woman, a palpable ovary may be a cyst, and should be watched over a four-to-six week period for signs of growth.

Again, what should a woman do if she has worrying symptoms? Any woman with persistent gastro-intestinal symptoms should not be fobbed off by her GP as suffering from middle-aged indigestion, or be told that it is all in her mind – if an examination/tests of the gastro-intestinal tract show that all is normal, a careful pelvic examination should follow, with other tests if necessary.

SCREENING FOR OVARIAN CANCER

At the time of writing, early screening for ovarian cancer is some years away, because no one knows what an ovarian 'pre-cancer' (the stage just before tissue turns cancerous) actually looks like. Various screening programmes are currently taking place to try to find out.

The ovarian screening programme at the London Hospital run by Dr Ann Prys Davies is screening high-risk women over the age of thirty-five, using a combination of three tests. The first is a blood test, to measure a substance called CA 125 (cancer antigen 125), which is higher in the blood of those women with ovarian cancer than in normal women. If the blood test is 'positive', the woman is recalled for two other tests: a bi-manual pelvic examination and an ultrasound scan. If the scan reveals an abnormality of the ovaries, appropriate treatment is arranged. Up to 30,000 women will be treated over a three-year period. A similar study is being done in Scandinavia.

None of the three tests is considered sufficient on its own. For example, ultrasound can pick up an abnormality, and although it can tell the difference between cancer and fibroids, it cannot tell the difference between a cyst and a cancer. Also, CA 125 testing can miss some early ovarian cancers. As a result, some women will need pelvic surgery to make a correct diagnosis, only to discover that they don't have cancer. One ovarian cancer screening specialist remarks, 'If we find a benign tumour then we still must operate – this is because we don't know what a pre-cancer looks like, and so we cannot just leave the tumour to see if it will turn malignant.'

However, there is constant hope for the improvement of diagnostic techniques. Research is under way on monoclonal antibodies (see p.44) and attempts are being made to sharpen the diagnostic abilities of ultrasound, which means that the 'false positive rate' (those women who may have ovarian cancer until surgery proves otherwise) is dropping all the time. It may never drop to zero, but this is the problem with a cancer that starts so deeply within a woman. To help the situation, screening technicians are being trained to recognise the appropriate-sized ovary for the appropriate age group.

Women who are eligible should take part in screening programmes, because at the moment this is all we have in the way of weapons to fight this sneaky, silent cancer. Only the results gathered from thousands of screening tests will reveal whether there is a test that can possibly diagnose ovarian cancer at an early stage, when it is possible to cure it. More advanced disease is much more difficult to treat, and much harder to cure.

If you would like to take part in the London Hospital screening programme, are over thirty-five and have a family history of ovarian cancer, contact Dr Ann Prys Davies at the London Hospital (see addresses). Women in the UK living outside London may find that their GP is taking part in this screening project, and he/she could enter you. The project is running for an indefinite period.

Another study that began in December 1989, hopes to collect together up to 1,000 women whose mother or whose mother and sister had ovarian cancer. The first stage will be a question-naire, and the second stage in 1990 will be a screening programme involving ultrasound, CA 125 and other tests. The screening will take place in six major cities in the UK, and a serum bank will be started to store the blood of high-risk women for the future development of better blood markers. The total programme will liaise with several European countries, and will run for an indefinite period. It is being funded by the Imperial Cancer Research Fund and the Royal College of Obstetricians and Gynaecologists. If you would like to take part contact Dr Peter Mason (see addresses).

The Imperial Cancer Research Fund Study is also screening women (for an indefinite period) who can claim a close relative with ovarian cancer, and more volunteers are needed here too. Contact Dr Tom Bourne at King's College Hospital, London (see addresses). This screening procedure begins with a vaginal ultrasound, which looks at the blood flow through the ovaries as a way of detecting tumour activity; and screening also includes abdominal ultrasound and a blood test.

It may be five years before all the results are in, and another five years before any kind of a reliable screening test can be set up nationally – but it could save an estimated 3,000 lives a year in the UK. Early results from the studies have been encouraging: in the King's College survey, seven out of 250 abnormalities picked up from ultrasound scans on 5,000 women over five years proved to be early-stage ovarian cancer. In the present King's College Hospital study of women with a family risk, four cases of stage 1 ovarian cancer were discovered among 650 women screened. The London Hospital study (which is generally screening women over forty-five) has picked up twelve ovarian cancers from 20,000 normal women who were screened. Says Dr Jacobs, 'If we could increase the proportion of diagnosed stage 1 cancer to three-quarters, we could perhaps improve the overall survival rate from 25 – 30 per cent to 60 – 70 per cent.

THE ORTHODOX FUTURE

The future for ovarian cancer involves better early screening and the creation of specific drugs to fight the disease which will be put 'on the backs' of 'designer' antibodies (like monoclonal antibodies, created in the laboratory for a specific purpose) capable of tracking down ovarian cancer in the body and in the bloodstream.

WHAT YOU CAN DO TO HELP YOURSELF

Follow this advice if you think you may be at risk:

- Use the contraceptive pill.
- Avoid talcum powder in the vaginal area.
- Have a bi-manual pelvic examination every year.
- Enrol yourself, as well as any female relatives, in a screening programme if you/they are over the age of forty-five or if your family has a history of ovarian cancer.
- Cut down on fats, as high fat consumption is thought to be linked to ovarian cancer.

THE COMPLEMENTARY APPROACH

Diet

Follow the 'anti-cancer' diet, or any of the diets given on pp.186 – 197. Ensure that any meat or poultry you may eat is hormone-free.

Vitamins

Take all the vitamins and enzymes mentioned on p.197, especially vitamins B6 and A. Vitamin A has been shown to cause regression in epithelial cancers like ovarian. Be very sparing with vitamin E, as large doses are linked to hormone activity (see p.203 for a suitable dosage).

Minerals

Take all the minerals mentioned on p.203, especially magnesium. Do not take any calcium supplements, as the receptor cells in ovarian cancer are tied up with calcium.

Supplements

Try gamma linoleic acid (GLA), bromelain or Iscador. Avoid ginseng, as it is a hormone stimulant (see p.210).

Herbal remedies

These are prescribed according to the individual patient's needs, but among herbs you may be treated with are Poke Root and Wild Yam to clean out the lymphatic system; also Wild Violet leaves, which herbalists believe to be cancer-inhibiting. The remedies are best taken as teas, but can also be taken as tincture drops, fluid extracts, tablets or capsules. (See pp.226 – 30.)

Homeopathy

Homoeopathic remedies are also presented according to the needs of the individual, and there are many for the homoeopath to choose from, but you may be given lycopodium, which is used to treat ovarian cysts so it may be helpful for other ovarian growths too. Remedies like nitric acid can also be prescribed to help with the side effects of chemotherapy (see p.233).

Other things you may want to try

These include acupuncture (p.239), counselling, relaxation, bio-feedback, breathing techniques (p.244), meditation, visualisation, and spiritual healing (p.250).

6
Cervical Cancer

The cervix is the lower, narrow part of the womb or uterus, at the top of the vagina. It is often referred to as the 'neck' of the womb. In the centre of the outer surface of the cervix is an opening called the 'external os', which leads to the narrow cervical canal, the passage through the cervix that connects the upper vagina with the main part of the uterus. It is through this passage that menstrual blood and glandular secretions pass, and leave the body via the vagina. The cervix lubricates the vagina for sex, and also helps the sperm to reach the egg during fertilisation.

The surface layer of the cervix consists of two different kinds of cells: flat or 'squamous' cells and more elongated ones called 'columnar' cells. The place where these two types of cells meet is called the transformation zone – and this is where abnormal cell changes can take place. A doctor can see and feel the cervix during an internal examination, and it is the cells in the transformation zone that are examined in a cervical smear test.

THE FACTS

- **UK incidence.** In 1984, 4,567 new cases were registered (4 per cent of all cancer registrations).
- **England and Wales five-year survival rate.** From 1981, 58 per cent of patients were alive five years later.
- **UK mortality.** In 1986, 2,234 patients died (3 per cent of all cancer deaths).

In England and Wales alone, between 4,000 and 5,000 women contract cervical cancer and 2,000 women die from it every year, and in some areas of England, the rate of cervical *pre*-cancer is increasing at an alarming rate. Worldwide there are 500,000 new cases diagnosed every year, with an epidemic in places like Africa and South America. In Africa, Central and South America, China, India and other Asian countries it is the most common female cancer. In North America and Europe it is the fourth most common cancer. In Australia cervical cancer accounts for 5 per cent of all cancer deaths. Overall, for women cervical cancer is the second most common cancer after breast cancer.

In general there has actually been a decrease in this disease: in developed countries mortality declined approximately 30 per cent between 1960 and 1980 as a result of screening and prompt treatment. The disease occurs at about the same rate in all women of ages above thirty, but there has been an increase in the thirty-five-and-under age group of 6 per cent in the last ten years. One in twenty deaths occur in women under the age of thirty-five.

Of all the four female cancers, cervical cancer has the strongest relationship with social class: it tends to hit the lower classes, who can't be reached as easily by doctors and the media, and it is more likely to kill off deprived white and black women alike, as well as women in the developing world. As one senior research registrar has remarked, often women who die from cervical cancer are those with little or no medical awareness, who would not have come in for a smear anyway. According to oncologist Tim Oliver, the husbands of these women probably had little knowledge of or access to basic hygiene facilities over twenty to thirty years ago when the seeds of the cancer were first initiated.

Cervical cancer is thought to be caused by a virus, and is probably not hormone-dependent in the way that the other three female cancers are. There are several DNA viruses which have been implicated including the papilloma (wart) virus, the *Herpes simplex* virus, the Epstein-Barr virus (thought to be the virus causing glandular fever) and the hepatitis virus. At the moment, the finger points most strongly at the wart virus.

There may be two kinds of cervical cancer: a slow-growing type with a detectable pre-invasive stage which is susceptible to treatment: and a more rapidly growing type which is harder to treat and which does not have a long pre-invasive stage. Some of the faster-growing cancers have been known to grow to the size of a football within four weeks, but fortunately these are relatively rare.

An established cancer doesn't shrink after the menopause (like fibroids) – if left untreated, most cases will continue to grow and spread. When it spreads, it does so along the lymphatic system rather than via the bloodstream. Fortunately, this cancer doesn't run in families in the same way that the other three female cancers do.

Unlike the other three cancers, cervical cancer has a clearly defined pre-cancerous stage, when the cells are in between being normal and cancerous. This stage is call 'cervical intra-epithelial neoplasia' ('CIN'). CIN is divided into three stages: CIN 1, where there are slight cell changes; CIN 2, where there are moderate cell changes; and CIN 3, where there are severe cell changes (see p.81 for more details). After CIN 3 there is a condition called 'carcinoma in situ', where the cancer cells are confined to the surface of the cervix and are not invasive – it is still considered part of CIN 3. 'Invasive cancer' is where cancerous cells grow deeper than the surface layer of the cervix and into other tissues.

SYMPTOMS

The symptoms of cervical cancer include abnormal bleeding, such as bleeding after sex or new bleeding in women who have had the menopause; offensive vaginal discharge, perhaps bloodstained; and abdominal pain. Even if a woman has had a negative smear, she should return to her GP if there is any abnormal bleeding.

RISK FACTORS

Statistical studies suggest that the following are possible risk factors for cervical cancer (they are not necessarily direct causes of the cancer): sexual activity, especially if your sex life started early; multiple sex partners for either the woman or her partner; a history of vaginal warts, especially in combination with vaginal herpes; a history of venereal disease, or of other sexually transmitted diseases; sexual hygiene of the male partner; occupation of the woman and of her partner (see page 75); having two or more children before the age of thirty; lack of vitamins; narcotics; and smoking, especially while taking the contraceptive pill. There is some evidence that stress may be connected, as it can lower the effectiveness of the immune system.

Using an intra-uterine contraceptive device does not increase the risk of getting cervical cancer, and neither does using tampons.

CIN makes a woman and her partner feel guilty, as if they are responsible for the disease. But the exact cause of CIN is unknown, and only a very small number of the women who have any of the known risk factors will develop CIN. It is also unfair to blame a woman's promiscuity, as many women who develop CIN have had only one sexual partner, in which case it may reflect on the number of sexual partners that the man has had. Or sexual relations may not be an accusative factor at all.

The woman who may be *most* at risk is the woman not in regular contact with her local health service or family planning clinic: this could be an older woman, with grown-up children.

The link with sexual activity

A joint study by the Imperial Cancer Research Fund, the University of Oxford and the John Radcliffe Infirmary in Oxford revealed that the risk of pre-cancer and carcinoma in situ among women who had their first sexual intercourse before the age of seventeen was two to three times higher than for women who started sex at twenty-one years and over. For the seventeen-to-eighteen-year age group, the risk was slightly less, and for the eighteen-to-nineteen-year-olds, it was less again. This may be because the cervixes of young women are still developing and are more vulnerable to the infections that seem to be linked to cervical cancer; young women are also more likely to use the pill than barrier methods of contraception, which are believed to offer protection against the disease (see p.75).

But the number of sexual partners is thought to be *more* important than a woman's age at first experiencing sex; and thought to be equally important is the number of sexual partners her spouse has had. If the male partner has had sex with any women with cervical abnormalities, he could pass on the cancer-inducing agents to his next partner. This is why women who have had only one partner can contract cervical cancer. Ninety per cent of cervical cancer originates in the exposed squamous cells of the cervix, which is why virgins do not get it, but virgins *can* contract another kind of cervical cancer called an 'adenocarcinoma', which arises from the epithelial lining of the cervix.

One research study suggests that frequent exposure of the cervix to the proteins in semen may lower a woman's defences against cancer. Unfortunately, this may be a biological necessity, as these proteins protect the sperm and enable them to avoid being rejected before they get to the egg. However, it is possible that the cumulative effect of the sperm of a number of different partners may heighten her risk of getting cervical cancer.

Wart virus and herpes virus

It isn't just semen which is the problem; it is what semen may be *carrying* – namely the wart virus, also known as human papilloma virus (HPV). It appears at the moment that there is a strong association between some members of the wart virus family, in either the woman or her partner, and the development of cervical cancer. It is not known whether the wart virus causes cancer on its own or is triggered into causing cancer when in the presence of other factors, or whether it is merely an 'assistant' to other cancer agents, in the way that the herpes virus is now thought to be an 'assistant' rather than a 'cause'.

Wart virus is a general term for a whole group of viruses (at least sixty) which cause warts in different parts of the body (and up to 80 per cent of the population may be carrying one form or another), but twelve have already been shown to be associated with cervical cancer. However, it must be clearly understood that it is not normally the genital wart virus which is associated with cervical cancer – the culprits are, in fact, other members of the wart virus family, related to the viruses which cause genital warts. The nasty-looking genital warts that you can see are usually not lethal; it is often the innocent-looking things that can be health-threatening – a thickening of the epithelium of the cervix, for example, may mean that a wart virus associated with cervical cancer has moved in. In almost all cases of advanced cervical cancer there is viral DNA present, derived from one of the culprit wart viruses (types 16, 18, 31 and 33 show up most often).

Wart virus could exist invisibly in a man's or a woman's genital tract, or exist on the cervix where only a doctor could see it. If your doctor finds visible warts, they will be treated, but if *you* spot them, you should get both yourself *and* your partner treated, in case he re-infects you: this is because genital warts have a nasty habit of recurring if only one cell is left, and can be unpleasant/embarrassing to experience; but, more importantly, there is a strong correlation between the presence of genital warts and the presence of other wart viruses which can cause pre-malignant or malignant lesions on the cervix. Genital warts are not bad in themselves, but they can be a warning sign, in the same way that a positive smear acts as a warning sign.

Lesions or 'warts' (caused by wart virus 6 or 11) can be treated in a variety of ways, all of which are painless to you, but harmful to the wart. They include freezing, burning, painting with a corrosive material or, more usually, laser surgery. Individual bouts of warts can be treated, never to return, although there is no permanent cure for wart virus yet.

With all the publicity given to it, HPV must be kept in perspective: out of 1,000 women only 100 will have HPV infection, and only one will go on to develop malignant cells. Dr Lionel Crawford, virologist, believes that the risk to women has been greatly exaggerated: it is not unusual to carry a member of the wart virus family in your system, even a malignant member; but carrying a malignant wart virus is not enough to make you contract cervical cancer. It is less than half the story, as many other factors are involved, some of which are not yet well understood. So, although it is wise to be aware of wart virus, it must be remembered that the vast majority of women with a malignant wart virus do not go on to develop cervical cancer – the reason for this appears to be that their immune system has managed to keep a 'lid' on it.

The herpes virus used to be considered a strong factor in

cervical cancer, but this is no longer the case. Recent studies haven't confirmed any link with cervical cancer and it may be that the virus's activity is very sideline, such as merely encouraging the wart virus, which itself needs other factors to make it a cancer-inducing agent.

Even if you have suffered from both wart virus and the herpes virus, don't panic: up to 70 per cent of women have no problem with either. But having both conditions does mean that you are entitled to an *annual* smear, and your GP should be agreeable to this.

Sexual infections

Sexually transmitted diseases, such a syphilis, gonorrhoea, candida, gardnerella, chlamydia and trichomoniasis may have an initiating role in causing cervical cancer. They may alter the genetic material of cervical cells in a series of steps, so it is always wise to have any genital irritation or infection treated promptly.

Sexual hygiene

Cervical cancer is less common in women married to circumcised men. Bacterial and viral carcinogens can become trapped under the penile foreskin, especially if a man has a dirty or dusty job – if he is a miner or has some other underground job, or is a metal, leather or textile worker, machinist, or an employee in a certain type of chemical factory. Female textile workers also have an increased incidence of cervical cancer. Many of the above male occupations also carry a high risk of cancer of the penis or of the scrotum.

It is clear that barrier methods of contraception are useful protection against cervical cancer. Oncologist Tim Oliver remarks, 'Men must learn that it's not 'sissy' to wash their penises, but rather that it will help protect their women against cervical cancer.' In one US study, of 139 patients with CIN who used a condom but received no medical treatment, 136 made a complete recovery. The study concluded that the women had had protection from viruses in the men's semen while their immune system recovered enough to fight the cancer off.

The number of children before thirty

Describing the number of children a women has before the age
of thirty as a risk factor in cervical cancer is misleading, because
the pregnancies themselves are not 'risky' – it is the possibility
of a torn cervix *resulting* from a pregnancy. The theory goes that
this might increase the risk by making necessary an excessive
growth of cervical epithelium to repair the damage, thus
reducing DNA repair time. In other words, the cells are kept
busy making scar tissue and so can't repair any DNA damage
as quickly as usual. The more full-term pregnancies, the higher
the chance that a tear might occur. The cervix of a woman
below the age of thirty is also more vulnerable because of the
higher level of hormonal activity it is undergoing. Clearly this
cervical cancer risk factor is at odds with the ovarian cancer
'avoidance tactic' of having children *before* the age of thirty. This
is because each cancer has different risk factors. Although all
risk factors should be kept in mind, they need to be taken with
a small dose of salt because 'apparent' risk factors are worked
out in a 'backwards' fashion: that is, for many risk factors,
doctors and scientists start with large groups of patients with a
particular female cancer and work back to factors they *appear* to
have in common (like having babies before the age of thirty).

Vitamin deficiencies

Studies of women with positive smears revealed that these
women took in less than 30 mg of vitamin C daily. It is not well
known that both smoking and the contraceptive pill can rob the
body of vitamin C. In another study of women with early cancer
of the cervix, there was found to be less beta-carotene (vitamin
A) in their bloodstream than in those women in the control
group. These particular vitamin deficiencies may or may not be
linked to cervical cancer: it could be that the cancer itself caused
the deficiency – either directly, or indirectly through
decreasing the appetite so that fewer foods containing these two
vitamins were eaten.

As vitamins A and C are known to be useful in cancer
prevention, however, it would be a good idea to make sure you
take in plenty of both (see Chapter 11). Folic acid, a B vitamin
important in the synthesis of DNA and RNA, seems to help

cervical pre-cancer: when it was given to a group of women with mild to moderate cervical dysplasia (abnormally developing cells), they did significantly better than the placebo group. Vegetables are a good source, if taken as a supplement, the suggested intake is 200 units a day.

Narcotics

Any drug that is used for an auto-immune disease such as rheumatoid arthritis, ulcerative colitis or thyroid disorders, could be a co-factor in cervical cancer. Heroin use weakens immunity in the same way that smoking weakens it.

The contraceptive pill

The contraceptive pill is not listed as a risk factor, although it seems to become one when linked with smoking. Generally, the link between the pill and cervical cancer, if any, is highly debatable. It may turn out that cervical cancer *is* hormone-dependent like the other three female cancers, in which case the pill would have an effect; or it may turn out to be a weak co-factor when used long term. But any risk from the contents of the pill is *so* slight that it is not worth stopping the pill for – particularly in view of how much protection the pill provides against ovarian cancer. The pill itself is not a carcinogen, but it is associated with a risk more because it allows 'risky' sexual behaviour, and is a substitute for more protective barrier contraception.

Smoking

A woman who smokes, or a non-smoking woman with a smoking partner, is more likely to develop cervical pre-cancer. Cigarettes contain one of the strongest known carcinogenic chemicals which, when inhaled, gets into the bloodstream and is then excreted in the urine. It may also be found in other body secretions, indicating that the body (including the cervix) become soaked in carcinogens. There is an additional factor linking smoking to cervical cancer, involving the body's Langerhans' cells. In a 1988 study undertaken by a group of British doctors and funded by various cancer research organisations, cigarette smoking was found to reduce the number of

Langerhans' cells. These cells fight infection and are that part of the immune system which specifically recognises viral infections and creates an immune response to them. So smoking can lower resistance in the cervix.

The more cigarettes smoked daily, the lower the Langerhan's cell count: smokers have half the cell count of those who have never smoked, and the cell count of ex-smokers falls somewhere between those of smokers and total abstainers. In one study, smoking twenty cigarettes a day was found to increase the risk of cervical pre-cancer by seven times. In an Australian study which has looked at 2,500 women over the last thirty years, more aggressive cervical cancer in younger women seems to be linked with smoking and sexual history.

The theory is that the effect of co-factors, such as smoking, on the immune system provides the trigger for progression to a pre-cancerous state. From these studies it would seem that not only can smoking expose the cervix to carcinogens which could mutate a benign growth into a more malignant one, but that smoking also reduces the body's resistance so that it is less able to reject the relevant virus in the first place. In fact, smoking is thought by many medical experts to impair the immune response very considerably, and drinking while smoking increases the risk as alcohol increases the absorption of the carcinogens in cigarette smoke.

DIAGNOSTIC TESTS

The cervical smear, or 'pap' test as it is sometimes called, is a simple screening test for cervical cancer and for those early cell changes that could lead to cancer. The importance of this test cannot be underestimated, as it can spot changes *before* symptoms appear. By the time symptoms appear, a tumour can be quite advanced. Ideally, sexually active women should have a smear test every year, and at *least* every three years. In 1986 four million smears were taken in the UK. It should have been 17.5 million, to cover all the women who need to have them, (see p.101 for the relation between the frequency of smear tests and the age of the woman).

A 'positive' smear test should be viewed only as a warning: at this stage there *isn't* any cancer, although the warning cells could *possibly* go on to develop into a cancer.

The smear test is similar to a vaginal examination, where you lie on a couch and a speculum is put gently into the vagina to dilate it. This allows the doctor to view the cervix. Then a spatula or brush is gently wiped across the cervix to take a sample of cells, after which the speculum is removed. The spatula is wiped across a slide which will be viewed under a microscope by a specially trained technician. The whole procedure is not painful, although you might find it uncomfortable if you are tensed up.

The smear test appears efficient at detecting a large number of abnormal cases – and because of the specific nature of the test, positive results are almost always reliable. But the smear test can miss up to 15 per cent of disease for the following reasons: if an inflammation, or thrush, is covering pre-cancerous or cancerous cells; if the tumour is high up in the cervical canal; or if someone inexperienced is doing the test, and cannot see the cervix to take a proper smear.

It is not enough just to make a microscope slide; the cervix must be *seen* by the doctor. A woman can ask her doctor during the smear test whether or not he/she can visualise the cervix properly.

Because there are up to 15 per cent 'false negative' results, many doctors argue strongly for annual screening. But as things stand now with the NHS, unless you have a history of herpes or wart virus it may be difficult to get screening more than once every three years. What tends to happen is that a smear is taken, and a second one follows in a year's time – if everything is all right, a smear will be taken every three years thereafter.

A woman should still be tested even after a hysterectomy, because although her cervix has been removed, it is still possible for pre-cancer or cancer to begin in the remaining tissue or vaginal skin. This is not actually a smear test, but a high vaginal swab. Other women should be aware of the difference between a smear test and a swab taken to detect sexually transmitted infections, which would be unable to detect pre-cancerous or cancerous changes.

There are four possible results of a smear test:

1. A normal (or 'negative') result;
2. Evidence of an infection or minor abnormality, which may or may not require treatment;

3.   Evidence of a pre-cancerous condition, called CIN;
4.   Evidence of a developed cancer.

Case Study – CERVICAL CANCER/HYSTERECTOMY

This story highlights the importance of insisting on a second opinion when you feel that there is something wrong with you, but your GP does not agree. It also points out the importance of having a smear test at least every three years – a five-year gap is too long, and could lead to a cancerous condition going undetected for several years.

Sue Southwood had gone for her five-year routine smear at the age of thirty-five and all had been well. At thirty-nine, one year away from her next five-year smear, she went to see her GP to complain about bleeding after sex and between periods. She was separated from her husband and there had been a two-year pause in her sex life before she met someone else.

Her doctor, whom she knew socially, assured her that it was just 'her age', and that she was fine. As Sue had just run a half-marathon, he proclaimed her to be fit. As an afterthought, however, he examined her cervix, but could see nothing wrong.

A month later, Sue's symptoms were no better. Her doctor's theory this time was that sex with her new boyfriend was slightly damaging her cervix, but this time he did a smear test. After a six-week wait the results returned 'normal' – but Sue's symptoms continued to get worse. Now her doctor's theory was that the contraceptive pill she had taken in her twenties had 'slightly eroded her cervix', but he agreed to send her to a specialist.

Sue had to wait two months for her 'non-urgent' appointment, at which she was kept waiting for two and a half hours before giving up. After walking out and realising that she would have to wait another three months for her next 'non-urgent' appointment, she decided to go privately. Having already booked a ski holiday, she waited until she was back before arranging an appointment with a specialist. Her only thought at this time was that she must be 'anaemic', and that her vegetarian diet must be a contributing factor.

It was March 1987 by the time she saw the specialist: a full year after she had first complained to her GP. A week later she was given a punch biopsy, and everything during this treatment 'looked' normal. But two weeks after this, when the sample was cultured, a very different message was telephoned through: she was borderline between CIN 3 and invasive cancer. Luckily, no lymph nodes appeared to be involved, and this was later confirmed by surgery. After a week of tests to check for spread, Sue had a hysterectomy. In the words of her surgeon, her growth had just started to move and to make satellite cells.

What had gone wrong? Sue did some investigating, and her training as a nurse and as a health visitor helped her. She discovered that her GP's method for taking a smear was outdated – he wasn't getting a total sweep of the cervix with the spatula during a smear take, and he didn't understand about the junction area on the cervix where cells could change. As a result, the lab had sent back her smear report as 'normal' when in fact it was a 'false negative'. She wrote to her Community Health Council and complained; they said that they would carry out their own investigation, but she heard nothing more.

She also told her GP how badly he had let her down, but he was mainly unrepentant. Surprisingly, she still sees him as her GP, because she feels that 'the devil she knows, is better than the devil she doesn't'. Not surprisingly, though, the relationship is now a cool one, with Sue telling her GP what she wants.

CIN

Cervical intra-epithelial neoplasia (CIN) simply means that when cervical cells are viewed under the microscope, they appear irregularly shaped or abnormal. It is in the 'transformation zone' of the cervix where columnar cells and squamous (flat) cells meet that abnormal cell changes can occur. Normally the softer columnar cells that find themselves facing outwards into the vagina are gradually changed into squamous cells, which are more suited for exposure to the outside world. This natural process is called 'squamous metaplasia'. If this is all that is happening, your smear will be 'negative'.

It is these changing cells, however, that could gradually, over a period of time, turn into cancer cells. Such rogue cells are called 'dysplastic'. At first the changes are slight, and this is known as 'mild dysplasia' or 'mild dyskaryosis' or CIN 1.

There is a condition called cervical erosion or 'ectophy', where the squamous cells are replaced by columnar cells on the surface of the cervix, making it appear inflamed. This condition is common, especially during puberty and pregnancy, or while on the pill, and it is *not* associated with CIN or cancer. It may sometimes cause bleeding or discharge, especially after sex, but it is harmless and can be easily treated.

If the cervical cells continue to change abnormally, though, they could become a 'moderate dysplasia' (or 'moderate dyskaryosis' or CIN 2). Or the cells could progress even further to a 'severe dysplasia' also known as 'severe dyskaryosis' or CIN 3. Your smear would be 'positive' as a result, but *none of these stages is cancer:* they are what is known as 'pre-cancer' (before cancer). These abnormal cells could, in time, turn cancerous, but the fact that there are a few abnormal cells in your smear doesn't mean that you will get cancer!

To summarise the *pre*-cancer state: CIN 1 involves only one-third of the thickness of the cervix's covering layer; CIN 2 involves only two-thirds of the thickness of the cervix's covering layer, and CIN 3 involves the full thickness of the cervix's covering layer.

To make things more complicated, diagnosticians may refer to classes 1, 2, 3, 4 and 5 which refer to the 'degree' of cell change present. Classes 1 and 2 refer to normal and inflammatory changes; class 3 can overlap between CIN 1 and CIN 2; class 4 can overlap between CIN 2 and CIN 3; and class 5 can overlap between CIN 3 and a 'carcinoma in situ'.

A 'carcinoma in situ' is where the cancer cells are confined to the surface tissue of the cervix and are *not* invasive, and it is still included in CIN 3. It is only when the abnormal cells penetrate *below* the surface layer of the cervix that true cancer of the cervix has developed.

One of the major problems with the government campaign started in March 1988 to give smear tests to all women between the ages of twenty and sixty-four is the lack of counselling about the differing degrees of cervical abnormality.

If you have CIN 1, a second smear will be done a few months later. If the second smear still shows the same result, you will be referred to a gynaecologist for a 'colposcopy'. Women with CIN 2 and CIN 3 will be referred immediately for a colpos-copy.

DIAGNOSTIC TESTS FOR CIN

Colposcopy

A colposcope is a special microscope on a stand that can take a closer look at the cervix. The smear test doesn't reveal everything, and a colposcope can show much further damage, if it exists.

The woman sits in a reclining chair, or lies on a table with her feet in stirrups, and a speculum is inserted to keep the vaginal walls apart. The gynaecologist, or 'colposcopist', shines a light on to the cervix, takes a smear test and then dabs the cervix with different liquids, such as saline, dilute acetic acid or iodine. The specialist then peers down the colposcope – the microscope does not go inside the woman. There might be a slight stinging sensation when the cervix is dabbed, or you might feel nothing at all. Abnormal cells show up as white; in some colposcopy clinics there is, attached to the colposcope, a closed-circuit television screen on which you may be able to see your own cervix. Or a photograph may be taken of your cervix as a record.

Punch biopsy

During colposcopy, the specialist might take a small sample of surface cervical tissue with biopsy forceps for further examination in a lab: this is called a 'punch biopsy'. It should be painless, although you might feel a slight nip. The specialist may be able to tell you then and there what degree of cell change is present, and even show you where the changed cells are by using a diagram or photograph, and specify a treatment. Or you may have to wait a few weeks for the lab test results on the punch biopsy. The whole procedure takes only ten to fifteen minutes.

Cone biopsy

A cone biopsy is used either to diagnose CIN more completely or to treat it.

Sometimes nothing can be seen through the colposcope, even though a woman's smears keep coming up positive. This would indicate that the abnormal cells are high up in the cervical

canal, an area that the colposcopist would be unable to see. This
can happen in older women, or in those women who have had
children. In this instance, a cone biopsy would be performed:
this involves the removal of a triangular wedge of the cervix
which contains the abnormal cells, with the point of the cone
extending into the cervical canal.

A cone biopsy is done under a general anaesthetic, and
requires a short stay of three to five days in the hospital. After
the operation, the tissue wedge is examined under a microscope. A small pack may be put into the vagina to prevent
bleeding, and is usually removed within twenty-four hours.
There may be some light bleeding after the operation which is
normal, and you will be advised to avoid sex and strenuous
physical activity for four weeks afterwards.

A cone biopsy cures 93 – 99 per cent of CIN 3 lesions, but
there are some drawbacks. The procedure can weaken the
cervical canal, which can then increase the risk of miscarriage
during pregnancy. If the cervical canal *is* weakened, a woman
can have a stitch put into the cervix to strengthen it during
pregnancy. If the cervix is badly scarred, a caesarian section
may be required when her baby is born.

Sometimes the sides of the cervical canal can tighten or
become narrower during the healing process as a result of scar
tissue: this is called 'cervical stenosis' and it can cause difficulty
with periods or during labour. It can affect 10 – 15 per cent of
women who have had a cone biopsy, so if your periods become
more painful after having one, notify your hospital doctor.

Case Study – CONE BIOPSY

*Roz Green had a cone biopsy in May 1989 at the age of thirty-five,
after having a smear with a 'severe abnormality' (CIN 3) in
January. She had never experienced a general anaesthetic before, but
found the whole procedure 'less traumatic' than the wait between the
smear and the cone biopsy. Roz had as large a cone as possible
removed, so that she wouldn't need to return for a second cone biopsy.
'The whole perimeter of the removed cone must be normal,' says
Roz, 'or it means that they haven't got it all.'*

*After the cone biopsy Roz found that she had bad period-type
pains, and she bled for seven weeks, heavily at first. Her first period
after the cone biopsy was also heavier and more painful than before.
The wadding inserted into her vagina after the operation, which is*

meant to dissolve gradually, had slipped downwards and pieces were leaving via the vagina for up to six weeks afterwards. (This can happen and does not indicate anything serious — it is more of an inconvenience). Physically it took Roz only two weeks to recover from the surgery, although mentally she felt fragile for longer. Despite the fact that she had made a conscious decision not to have any children, she was annoyed that no one had told her that a cone biopsy might affect her ability to carry a child.

Cervicography

Colposcopy is not widely available on the NHS because both the equipment and the training of specialists are expensive. Cervicography is used when there are no skilled personnel present to do an immediate colposcopy. A 'cervicograph' is a camera with a light source on the front of it, which can illuminate and photograph the cervix. The photograph is sent for examination to a specialist, who then recalls a patient for colposcopy, biopsy and treatment, if needed. The accuracy of cervicography is high: however, on the one hand, it can pick up some 'false positives', while on the other, it can miss some abnormalities in the cervical canal.

Cervicography is useful with recurring cervical lesions, because the surgeon can compare photographs of the cervix at various time intervals to pinpoint where the lesion is. The technique still needs further evaluation, though, and it won't be replacing colposcopy. A colposcopy is still essential to take biopsies, and to establish a diagnosis and a treatment.

The Schiller test

The Schiller test may be used when colposcopy is not available. It involves the application of iodine to the cervix: the normal areas are darkened by the iodine, while the abnormal parts are not darkened by it.

Examination under anaesthetic (EUA) and dilatation and curettage (D and C)

EUA and D and C are done when the suspected abnormal cells are out of range. Under a short, general anaesthetic where the abdomen is completely relaxed, the doctor can more easily examine the cervix and other organs. The doctor can then stretch the cervix enough (dilatation) to take a sample of cells (curettage) for examination. The patient is out of hospital the next day, with slight bleeding for a few days afterwards. If the bleeding is excessive, she should tell her doctor.

This technique can also be used to take a biopsy before surgery for cervical cancer, or before radiotherapy treatment, which is sometimes used instead of surgery. The surgeon can discover how far the cancer has spread, and he/she can do a more complete examination of the patient under anaesthetic without hurting her. When the abdomen is relaxed, the surgeon can tell if the cancer is mobile or fixed, and where the best place would be to make a surgical incision.

TREATMENTS FOR CIN

The main treatments for CIN are cone biopsy, laser therapy, diathermy, cryotherapy and cold coagulation. Sometimes when a woman is past her child-bearing years depending on the type of cervical cancer, the probability of recurrence, and the individual woman's situation and wishes, a hysterectomy (removal of the womb) might be suggested, but it is obviously better if a woman can avoid such drastic measures.

Laser therapy

Laser therapy is the ideal treatment for CIN because there is no cutting, and therefore no blood let loose to risk the spread of the disease. Its availability is limited on the NHS because of the expense, but if a hospital has a laser, its first line of treatment will usually be laser therapy. It involves the vaporisation of abnormal cells by a very intense beam of laser light under microscope (colposcope) control. Normal cells are left untouched.

Although there is a slight burning smell during the procedure, there is no pain, which means that it can be performed on an outpatient basis without a general anaesthetic. A local anaesthetic is used to prevent any discomfort. Afterwards, there may be some light bleeding and discharge, although the majority of women have no side effects at all. If the bleeding gets heavier, contact your GP or the outpatient department where you had treatment. Within six weeks new cells will have replaced dead ones and the cervix will be back to normal. The cervix heals rapidly after laser treament.

After treatment, there is a 95 – 97 per cent chance of a complete recovery; rarely is a second laser treatment necessary. A woman just needs to continue having regular smears. Laser therapy does not affect fertility or present a problem in pregnancy.

Case Study – LASER THERAPY

Rita Ferris-Taylor was thirty years old when, in August 1986, she had laser treatment for CIN 3. A local anaesthetic was injected into her cervix to take a small sample (punch biopsy), and a dye painted on the cervix to show up the area of abnormality. Rita found the punch biopsy, which lasted only a few minutes, more painful ('like being pinched') than the laser therapy. In fact she wasn't sure when the laser treatment started or stopped (there was no television screen in her hospital to view the laser procedure, as there is in some other hospitals). She could smell a burning smell, however, which lasted about five minutes. Afterwards Rita experienced a lot of heavy bleeding for about three weeks. Unfortunately she developed an infection which her GP treated with antibiotics. She had to wait a month before resuming sex, but everything was fine.

It wasn't until her next colposcopy in December 1986, which revealed everything to be 'normal', that Rita felt completely over the experience. She now has three-yearly smears.

Rita was happy about having laser therapy, because she knew it was the 'least invasive' of the treatment options and that it wouldn't cause scar tissue. Three months after her treatment Rita became pregnant and went on to have a normal delivery and a healthy baby – her cervix had not been damaged in any way.

Diathermy

Diathermy is done under a general anaesthetic (thus requiring an overnight stay in hospital) and involves the removal of abnormal cells by passing a tiny electric current through the affected area. It is used when CIN is severe or can't be reached by a laser. The procedure takes less than an hour, and there may be a slight vaginal discharge or light bleeding for a few days or weeks after treatment. There is a high rate of eradication of abnormal cells with only one treatment – some say up to 97 per cent.

A new type of diathermy involves a large loop excision of the transformation zone, which removes rather than destroys abnormal tissue and can be performed very quickly under a local anaesthetic. There is an increased risk of stenosis of the cervical canal (see p.84) with diathermy, making future cervical smears slightly more difficult to obtain, but the high success rate still makes it a worthwhile technique.

Cryotherapy

Cryotherapy (also known as cryosurgery or cryocautery) entails a small probe being placed on the surface of the cervix which freezes the abnormal cells through the application of liquid nitrogen or carbon dioxide. It is used to treat CIN 1 or 2 and can be performed in an outpatients' department. During treatment you may feel a mild, period-type pain, headache, dryness, nausea or hot flushing sensation, but this will disappear when the treatment finishes. Afterwards there may be a watery discharge for two to four weeks, which could be heavy at first, and sometimes there are strong, period-type pains immediately afterwards. If you experience any heavy bleeding as a result of the treatment, tell the doctor involved. The whole procedure takes about fifteen minutes. It is a slower, gentler treatment than laser therapy, but is not quite as accurate: the success rate with *one* treatment varies between 80 and 90 per cent.

Case Study – CRYOTHERAPY/CONE BIOPSY

Donna Franceschild was twenty-seven when her cervical smear was diagnosed as 'suspicious' in August 1980, and was asked to return for a repeat smear. Before this could be arranged however, she began to bleed. She had a history of cervical erosion and infections that would linger, and nine months previously she had experienced bleeding during sex.

In December 1980 Donna was treated with cryotherapy. She describes it as starting off much like a colposcopy, lying on a table with her feet in stirrups. For a few minutes it was painful, as cold gas was blown at her cervix. During the following two weeks she had a watery discharge.

Unfortunately for Donna she began to bleed again from the cervix, and a colposcopy confirmed 'carcinoma in situ', or, as it was explained to her, the middle stage between simple dysplasia and cancer. The specialist recommended a cone biopsy and quite a large cone was taken, which resulted in heavy bleeding afterwards. Because of the packing put into her vagina to stop the bleeding, Donna needed a catheter for two days.

The day after her hospital discharge she began to haemorrhage again, and so was taken back into hospital for more packing and a catheter. She was in for a total of ten days. Donna took things easy after this, avoiding sex for six weeks. She continued to have abnormal smears for a while which then returned to normal. As some mucous glands were taken during the operation, it is difficult for sperm to get into her cervix, and so pregnancy could be harder to achieve. There is also the danger of an 'incompetent cervix' as a result of the cone biopsy, making a cervical stitch necessary to keep a pregnancy safe.

Cold coagulation

Contrary to its name, this treatment involves *heat*, not cold, although a much cooler temperature is involved that that in diathermy. A heated probe is put on to the surface of the cervix, which burns the abnormal cells in less than two minutes. No anaesthetic is required as you won't feel this, although you may have a mild period-type pain during treatment. After treatment, there may be light bleeding for a few days. It is used less often than other methods, when the condition is not so severe. There are, however, reports of a 95 per cent cure with one treatment for CIN 3.

Laser therapy, cryotherapy and cold coagulation are all given on an outpatient basis, but take someone with you to help you home, as you may feel slightly wobbly or unwell after treatment. Both cone biopsy and diathermy require an anaesthetic, and so a short hospital stay is involved.

The success of CIN treatment

You will know within a few days of your chosen treatment if the treatment has been successful or not. If it hasn't been completely successful, another treatment will be recommended. You must carry on having regular smears after all the treatment is finished.

THE DIAGNOSIS

There are no tests which can predict the rate of progression from a pre-cancer to a cancer in the 30 per cent of CIN patients where this will happen – the rate varies with each individual, and could be anything from one to ten years. A cancer would be diagnosed after a smear test and colposcopy, or after the additional diagnostic tests of cone biopsy and/or EUA. There may also be blood tests, a chest X-ray, lymphogram, intravenous urogram (IVU) and a CAT scan to check on cancer spread. The IVU and the lymphogram are necessary to see if there is any blockage of the urinary system, or if there is lymph node involvement, both of which could render the tumour inoperable.

A few women may be offered nuclear magnetic resonance (NMR) in place of a CAT scan. NMR is a scanning device which uses strong magnetic waves to differentiate tumour from normal tissue. A picture is created which is projected on to a television screen. NMR is preferable to a CAT scan because it doesn't use radiation, although it hasn't yet been proved a superior technique – and neither technique can pick up a tumour less than 2 cm (0.75 inch) in diameter. NMR is expensive and therefore available in only a few hospitals.

TREATMENTS

Treatment of cervical cancer will depend on many factors, including a woman's age and general health, and the tumour's type, size and degree of spread. The first invasive stage of cancer, following after CIN 3 (also known as 'stage zero') is the micro-invasive stage, or 'stage 1', where the cancer cells dip below the surface layer of the cervix. A cone biopsy may get all the cancer, otherwise a hysterectomy (removal of the womb) may be necessary.

In 'stage 1', the tumour is still confined to the cervix: it can be treated by hysterectomy, or radiotherapy, with an 80 per cent chance of cure. In 'stage 2', the tumour has spread to the vagina and to the side of the cervix and neighbouring tissue; in 'stage 3', the tumour extends to the pelvic wall; and in 'stage 4', the tumour generally extends beyond the pelvis. Stages 2 to 4 are treated with radiotherapy, with a 60 per cent cure rate for stage 2, a 30 per cent cure rate for stage 3, and a 10 per cent cure rate for stage 4. Chemotherapy is not very effective against cervical cancer, particularly if the cancer has spread, but recent trials with the cytotoxic drug ifosfamide, the platinum drugs and a combination of drugs are showing encouraging results.

SURGERY

How much tissue is removed during surgery (see p.35 for a general introduction) depends on the depth of the invasion and the stage of the cancer. The surgeon may remove just the uterus (this operation is known as a hysterectomy), or the uterus with a small part of the vagina and some lymph nodes, or he/she may remove the uterus with the ovaries and the Fallopian tubes and lymph nodes (radical hysterectomy or hysterectomy and bilateral salpingo-oophorectomy). A Wertheim's hysterectomy removes the uterus, Fallopian tubes, ovaries (though these are sometimes left), lymph nodes and the top one-third of the vagina, and as a result is a much longer operation (see the case study on p.92). The surgeon must work more slowly to avoid damage to the bladder and ureters. Surgeons are now trying to save the ovaries in younger women, as 'squamous carcinoma', which accounts for 90 per cent of cervical cancers, is not hormone-sensitive and rarely spreads to the ovaries. Similarly, a young woman with a non-invasive cancer who aims to have children may be able to delay surgery with careful planning of her treatment.

The ligaments and muscles which support the female organs may also be removed in a hysterectomy if they have been affected. Most hysterectomies are performed by making either a horizontal (or transverse) cut in the abdomen, but occasionally the uterus can be removed via the vagina – in this case, the cut is internal, and there is no visible scar. Sometimes a vertical cut is needed for a radical hysterectomy, depending on how extensive the operation is. Discuss with your doctor what the possibilities are for you.

There can be complications with surgery, including damage

to the bladder and the urinary tract, which require further treatment, but this is uncommon.

After a hysterectomy, there will be a drainage tube from the wound for forty-eight hours to stop any excess fluid from collecting. However, if any lymph nodes have been removed, drainage tubes may need to remain in place for up to ten days. Sometimes a small tube (or catheter) is put into the bladder for a short time to allow the urine to drain while the bladder is healing. You may also need an intravenous drip of fluids and salts until you are able to eat and drink again (i.e. until the affects of the anaesthetic have worn off). The doctor and nurses will encourage you to start moving about as soon as possible, as this is an important part of your recovery. Even while you are still in bed, you will be persuaded to do leg movements and deep-breathing exercises!

There will be some pain after surgery while the incision is healing – there may also be pain from wind temporarily trapped in the bowel. Painkillers will be given throughout the post-operative period, but let your nurse know how much pain relief you need, and for how long.

You will be able to return home one to two weeks after your operation, once the stitches or clips have been removed. There will be a slight discharge or bleeding from the vagina similar to a light period for several weeks after surgery while internal healing is still taking place, and this is quite normal. Once at home, avoid any strenuous physical activity – especially heavy lifting – for about three months. Climbing stairs will be a problem for a while, so if you live alone, let the ward sister know so that help can be arranged.

The post-operative check-up takes place at the hospital's outpatient clinic: this is a good time to discuss with your hospital doctor any post-operative problems that you may be having, and to ask him/her how your recovery can be expected to go.

Case Study – WERTHEIM'S HYSTERECTOMY

Sheena Shaw was thirty-one when in March 1988 she had a Wertheim's hysterectomy for cervical cancer, discovered while she was having routine fertility tests. She'd had no previous symptoms and was devastated by the diagnosis as she and her husband had badly wanted children. Still, she was determined to recover from the operation as quickly as possible so that they could start adoption procedures.

She developed the hot flushes often associated with the menopause soon after the operation, and was given hormone replacement therapy (HRT) straight away. Although not an avid pill taker, Sheena was convinced by her GP of the long-term benefits of taking HRT. She also developed a slight bladder infection from the catheter, which was a normal reaction and quickly dispensed with by antibiotics.

She was told by her specialist to rest and not to do anything physical for six weeks. Just before her six-week check-up she was advised to try gentle sexual intercourse with her husband to see if there were any major problems (after a Wertheim's hysterectomy you need to make love more carefully until the newly shortened vagina becomes stretched again). At first Sheena found sex 'not quite the same', but this feeling disappeared over a period of time.

It took her three months to feel completely physically fit, although it was another three months before all the internal healing was completed, because there was some granulated tissue at the top of the vagina.

It was around the third month that the emotional implications of the procedure hit Sheena, and it took her several months to work through her grief and to the acceptance of a 'new me'. Her husband had feelings of guilt that he had caused her problem – but the doctor assured them both that sexual intercourse was not the cause, as no wart virus had been found (see p. 73).

Her vagina is now very dry, but Sheena counteracts this with KY Jelly. Her advice to women experiencing the same procedure is 'to take each day as it comes' and not to be a planner, which she tended to be. Also, Sheena feels strongly that 'full explanations' (of the operation) are not for everyone, but that such information should be made available if requested.

Case Study – RARE CERVICAL CANCER/ EARLY HYSTERECTOMY

Laura Court was twenty-four when she experienced sharp pain and bleeding during sex. This was in April 1986, and she'd had a smear test two and a half years earlier. Thinking it was thrush, she saw her doctor, who examined her and took a smear. Two weeks later the local hospital rang to ask her to come in for a colposcopy, during which a small sample of growth was taken. The results were back four days later: a rare kind of cervical cancer, apparently brought on by her mother taking a hormone drug to avoid miscarriage while pregnant with Laura. (Between the 1940s and the 1960s, millions of women took an oestrogen drug called DES during pregnancy to prevent miscarriage. Over 200 cases of a rare vaginal or a rare cervical cancer have been found in the daughters of these women). Laura never told her mother: 'I didn't want to worry her, as I knew she would only blame herself.'

Laura was referred to a cervical cancer specialist at a large hospital. Three weeks later she had a hysterectomy. Because her bladder had been bruised during the operation, Laura had to wear a catheter and bag for two months: the catheter tube came out of a small plastic disc which was fitted to the skin of her left groin, and the bag was strapped to the outside of her thigh. Apart from this inconvenient reminder of the operation, Laura was initially too busy 'getting better' to feel any immediate after-effects. Five months later, however, it suddenly hit her that she would never be able to have children. Her husband, too, was in a mild state of shock – being a scout leader and loving children, it took him time to adjust to the idea of not being able to have any of his own.

The radical hysterectomy had taken Laura's uterus, Fallopian tubes, 1 – 2 cm (0.5 inch) at the top of her vagina and some lymph nodes, but had left her ovaries. The lymph nodes turned out to be cancer-free. The only complication that Laura experienced apart from the catheter was a trapped lymph node in her groin – after a year of trying various painkillers and ultrasound, she was finally referred to a pain clinic where a course of three steroid injections finally left her free of pain from the lymph node.

Laura's vagina did tighten up after the hysterectomy, and while KY Jelly helped her, a dilator did not. Otherwise, she found that when she felt up to sex again, it was no different from before.

Both Laura's husband and parents were worried about her long-term prospects for survival. Laura herself felt as if she were on 'automatic pilot', but a check-up eight weeks after the operation, and then every six months since, has revealed everything to be fine.

Case Study – HORMONE REPLACEMENT THERAPY

Sue Southwood was put on hormone replacement therapy (HRT) six weeks after her hysterectomy to ease the menopausal symptoms brought on by her operation. She is on oestrogen only – she doesn't need progesterone as well because, without a womb, she's in no danger of endometrial cancer. At first her hormones were 'all over the place' and her symptoms included panic attacks and occasional hot *flushes. Her HRT 'patches', placed on the skin just above the buttock, seem to work better in summer than in winter, and have succeeded only in reducing her symptoms. Sometimes she feels as though she is not functioning well; she feels 'different', and food tastes 'different'. But Sue soon managed to return to an active lifestyle that includes weight-training, running and teaching aerobics.*

It took Sue about a year to feel 'normal' again, which is the average recovery time after a hysterectomy. Unfortunately but understandably, Sue's physical and emotional traumas put her off sex for a while, and her new relationship didn't survive the strain.

Sue's nearest support group was 24 km (15 miles) away, so she formed her own, with the help of two other women who had experienced hysterectomy. They call it 'Women to Women'. Sue counsels for the group, giving advice to women with gynaecological problems and positive smears, and also to those facing a hysterectomy.

Women have many anxious questions to ask Sue about the operation: 'How will I feel afterwards?'; 'What will I be able to do?'; 'What will sex be like?'; 'When will I be "normal" again?' Sue advises these women that they will start to feel better within two months of their operation, that they should get plenty of rest, and that lifting and pushing will be more difficult.

Sue emphasises the importance of HRT for getting back to normal, and counters the fear of further cancer – which is very small indeed with HRT – by saying that women who aren't on HRT get cancer as well. After her own experience, she recommends a smear test every three years, and she feels that the best people for this job are female doctors at the Family Planning Clinics, who are trained by the Family Planning Association and go on regular refresher courses. According to Sue, many GPs learn about smear-taking only by 'watching'. Says Sue: 'If a woman has any worries, she should ask questions – for instance, during a smear test, she could ask the doctor what her cervix looks like.'

Sue believes strongly in counselling for both the woman and her partner before the hysterectomy: 'It is essential to prepare a couple for what's to come. Sexual health relies on an understanding partner, as you feel different about your body afterwards and unsure about what you can do. A woman should speak to other women about hysterectomy, and continuing support should be there if she needs it.'

RADIOTHERAPY

The planning of radiotherapy treatment is individual to each patient and should be discussed carefully with your doctor and radiotherapist before treatment starts, particularly if there is any risk of permanent side effects. (See p.36 for general introduction to radiotherapy.) You may experience any of the following temporary side effects during treatment, but there are things that you can do to help yourself:

1. **Greater fatigue.** Get more rest.
2. **Nausea.** Anti-nausea drugs can be prescribed, or try eating little and often, avoiding greasy and highly spiced foods, drinking more fluids and avoiding alcohol.
3. **Diarrhoea.** Avoid green vegetables, fruit, bran and wholemeal products, and drink more fluids. Certain medications may help too.
4. **A mild sunburn on the skin between the groins and buttocks.** Lukewarm baths without soap or oil will help, but don't apply any cream unless the doctor has prescribed it.
5. **Slight burning on urinating.** Drink plenty of fluids, but if the problem persists, tell the nurse or doctor so that medication can be given.

When your treatment stops, the normal cells should repair themselves, and your body return to normal. There could be some permanent side effects, though, especially if the ovaries have been irradiated, such as an early menopause or scarring and drying of the vagina that may interfere with sexual intercourse. This is partly due to radiation treatment and partly due to the loss of oestrogen (if the ovaries stop working) which can cause the vagina to shrink and stiffen. This is why it is important to resume sex as soon as possible after radiotherapy, to keep the vagina 'in shape' and prevent sex from being difficult later.

Symptoms of an early menopause include hot flushes, dry skin, feelings of anxiety and depression, and loss of interest in sex. Hormone replacement therapy (HRT), in the form of tablets and/or cream, will ease any symptoms.

The internal organs (vagina, ovaries, bowel, bladder) are

shielded as much as possible during treatment, but sometimes not with complete success. In a very small percentage of women (2 – 6 per cent), depending on age, individual reaction to surgery and the extent of the surgery, there may be 'radiation cystitis' (frequent emptying of the bladder), 'radiation enteritis' (narrowing of the rectum) or intermittent diarrhoea. The bowel problems can be controlled by a low-fat/low-fibre diet and by tablets.

Internal radiotherapy

This technique is being used less and less. It involves putting a small radioactive implant – rods of caesium in a tube – into the womb to fight the cancer from the *inside*. The dose is a small one, but for the few days that the implant is in, you will need to be nursed in a separate room, possibly behind lead shields. This is to keep the dose to a minimum for visitors and nurses. Visitors will be restricted, and children will not be encouraged to visit during this time.

You will feel isolated during the treatment, but once the implant is removed, all the radioactivity disappears. You will need to lie very still in bed to help the treatment along, and you may have a catheter in your bladder to help with the extra flow of urine that the radioactivity creates. You will be encouraged to eat healthily and to drink lots of fluids during treatment. Any side effects can be treated with tablets, but treatment can narrow the vagina. A woman should be told that this may happen, and afterwards given dilators and KY Jelly to help her should such vaginal narrowing occur.

Case Study – RADIATION IMPLANT
Pauline Hislop was thirty-eight when she was given internal radiotherapy as a way to reduce the size of her cervical cancer tumour before surgery.

Under a general anaesthetic, a radioactive implant was put into her vagina – it only took a few minutes. Pauline describes it as being like a solid metal cigar, 15 × 5 cm (6 × 2 inches). She was then put in a four-bed ward. As the radiation from the implant was emitted only from the sides of the body, Pauline was allowed to have visitors as long as they stayed at the foot of her bed.

Pauline had the implant in for five days, and she found it 'uncomfortable, like having bad period pains', although she was given painkillers to help. She also felt restricted in her movements, because of the catheter for her bladder which was necessary so that she could stay in bed.

After five days an instrument was hooked to the end of the implant to pull it out. Removal was the most painful part. A simulator then measured where the radiation had reached.

Pauline was encouraged to drink lots of water afterwards (slowly) to flush any remaining radiation out through her urine. The hospital ensured she was able to pass urine on her own (after they removed the catheter) before she was allowed to go home. She was home from this procedure in a matter of hours.

Pauline received her treatment in 1985, and some hospitals are now administering internal radiotherapy by different means.

SURVIVAL TIMES

Survival time is linked to the overall stage and grade of the tumour, how much tumour is left after surgery and whether there has been any spread to the lymph nodes. If the lymph nodes nearest the tumour are clear of cancer, there is only a 10 per cent chance of recurrence. The number of nodes involved can proportionately reduce survival time: one to four nodes involved can mean *on average* that 50 per cent of patients survive five years; and five or more nodes involved can mean on average that less than 20 per cent of patients survive five years. However, if a woman gets past the crucial 'five years', she should be fine, because a relapse very rarely occurs after this time with this cancer.

CIN HELP

CancerLink, one of the cancer help organisations, receives a lot of phone calls from women with positive smears who think that they have cancer. It cannot be emphasised too strongly that a smear that comes back 'positive' with signs of CIN is *not* cancer. But how many cases of CIN, if left untreated, *do* go on to develop into cancer? Somewhere around 30 per cent, although a New Zealand doctor's research put it as high as 50 per cent. The problem is that no one can be sure *which* patients would be in the cancer percentage.

About one-third of CIN 1 (and some CIN 2) cases disappear by themselves, leaving one-third or less of cases remaining stable. CIN 3 is unlikely to disappear by itself. On average CIN doesn't become invasive for eight to ten years, and sometimes it takes as long as fifteen years. After one year, only 4 per cent of the 30 per cent will have developed an invasive cancer; after three years, 11 per cent; after five years, 22 per cent; and after nine years, around 30 per cent. Severe lesions move much more quickly, and many cervical cancers do not follow an orderly development: they can appear as a CIN 2 or a CIN 3, or develop to an invasive cancer *without* a CIN stage.

Some women feel 'diseased' or 'tainted', especially as the abnormal cells are hidden in a sexual area. A supportive and understanding partner can make all the difference – don't let a few abnormal cells come between you! Once the unhealthy cells are removed, a healthy new layer of tissue grows over the whole transformation zone. If you are worried about whether you can have sex with CIN, ask your doctor: with a mild pre-cancer, it should be OK, although a condom will be recommended for your partner to protect your cervix against further damage. After CIN treatment, you will need to wait three to four weeks for the area to heal before resuming sex. The cervix heals well after treatment for CIN.

Another worry for women with CIN is whether it will happen again. The development of abnormal cells probably results from several factors coming together at the same time, with something triggering off the growth. The same combination of factors is unlikely to happen again, but if it does, subsequent smears will pick this up and it can be treated in the same way as before.

Another fear that women express is whether they can get pregnant after CIN, particularly after a cone biopsy – and the answer is yes. The treatment for CIN does not affect your sex life or your ability to get pregnant – excluding hysterectomy, of course, which is rarely used as a CIN treatment.

PREGNANCY AND ADVANCED CIN/CERVICAL CANCER

But advanced CIN/cervical cancers do present problems when they are discovered *during* a pregnancy. CIN 3 occurs in approximately one in 500 pregnancies in Britain; invasive cancer occurs in one in 20,000 pregnancies. Orthodox treatment depends upon when the invasive lesion is diagnosed: if it is during the first trimester of pregnancy, treatment would in itself cause an abortion. Treatment would consist of external radiotherapy, followed by internal radiotherapy, followed by a hysterectomy if necessary.

If advanced CIN/cervical cancer were discovered in the second trimester of pregnancy, the foetus would be delivered by hysterectomy, which would be followed by external and internal radiotherapy and, if necessary, surgery. If disease is discovered in the last trimester, treatment would be delayed until the baby was delivered by a caesarian section, then treatment would be the same as for the second trimester.

FEAR ABOUT THE SMEAR

It is the negative media hype that has given many women the wrong impression about cervical cancer and the smear test. The term 'cancer smear' conjures up the idea of cancer straight away – so that when some women are told that their smears are 'positive', they believe that they already have a fatal illness.

When research was done to find out why more women don't go for smear testing, it was revealed that fear of the test itself was a major hurdle. Those older women in the study who thought that the causes of cervical cancer were due to a 'germ', smoking or a 'shock' believed the test to be painful and embarrassing. Oddly enough, the younger women in the study who thought cervical cancer was caused by promiscuity, early sex or the contraceptive pill believed more in the validity of the test. Many older women did not like the idea of an internal investigation, even if they had had children, believing that that part of their body was 'finished with'.

Some older and younger women alike in the study regarded cervical cancer as a 'dirty disease', contracted by promiscuous women, and that to go for the test was tantamount to being tarred with the same brush.

The research mentioned here was undertaken by consultant psychologist Jennifer King in 1986, on women aged thirty-five and over, representing a range of social classes in four health centres in Oxford. The result of the research was to encourage local GPs to send out letters to their female patients explaining the benefits of the smear test, and informing them out of their misconceptions: that the test was painless and that a positive result generally didn't mean cancer but only signified the presence of abnormal cells which could be removed by a simple procedure. The letter would also point out that a woman could have a female GP or nurse to do the test if that was preferable, and that the test was just as important for women over forty-five as for those over thirty-five. In effect, this 'ideal' GP's letter would cover all the reasons why women did not go for smear testing.

Where to go for a smear test

Every woman who is sexually active should go for regular smear tests, and she should go for her first test within five years of starting sex. If the first test has not been performed before the age of thirty, it should be repeated within a year to confirm that it is 'negative' – after that, the test should be performed annually if there are risk factors, and every three years if there are not.

Women who have had CIN will be tested every six months for two years, and then annually. You can stop having smears between the ages of sixty-five to seventy, provided that the last two smears were negative and there is no history of doubtful or positive smears. This does not apply to women who have had a hysterectomy for a benign lesion: for them, testing would finish with the surgery.

In April 1988 the government began a computer-controlled national cervical screening programme. Women aged twenty to sixty-four were invited to attend various centres for a cervical smear at least every five years (three in some cases). The system, called the 'Call/Recall Programme', is working better in some areas of the country than others, so contact your local Family Practitioner Committee (listed in the telephone directory) for more information. Smears can also be taken by your GP, a family planning clinic, a well woman clinic or an STD (sexually transmitted diseases) clinic. By the way, you don't need a sexually transmitted disease to attend an STD clinic! The Women's National Cancer Control Campaign (WNCCC) will also have details of screening in your area (see the list of addresses on p.278).

Make an appointment for a test when you know you will not have a period. It can take several weeks to get the results back, but to avoid them being lost in the post, leave a self-addressed stamped envelope with the testing centre and ask them to notify you *one way or the other*. No news is not necessarily good news. If abnormal cells are present in your smear, contact your GP, who will arrange either for a second smear test or a referral on to a gynaecologist.

THE ORTHODOX FUTURE

The future for cervical cancer involves the development of many factors on the preventative, diagnostic and treatment levels, and includes the following:

- The possible development of a blood test as an early warning device.
- The possible development of a vaccine against the papilloma wart virus.
- Educating young men about the importance of genital hygiene.
- Automating screening procedures and increasing the sensitivity of the smear test to provide more reliable smear results.
- The development of a means of assessing which CIN cases are potentially invasive.
- The further development of interferon, interleukin, photo-chemical therapy and better chemotherapy as potential treatments.

If it turns out that hormones play a similar role in encouraging cervical cancer to that which they play in breast cancer, there may one day be an 'early warning' blood test, which would be used in conjunction with specific drugs to prevent the cancer – although some doctors believe this to be unlikely. Until then, the cervical smear remains the main diagnostic technique.

Dr Lionel Crawford, under the auspices of the Imperial Cancer Research Fund, is seeking to devise a vaccine against the wart virus (HPV). The approach will be two-fold: first, to vaccinate all girls before they reach the age of puberty; and second, to boost the immune system in the cervix itself by vaccinating women from their late teens to their early fifties after they have been found to have HPV infection, where cells are pre-malignant but not yet cancerous. The first approach is considered impractical by some doctors for reasons of social acceptability and the sheer numbers involved. The second approach would aim to lengthen the time between a woman's becoming infected with HPV and her developing pre-cancerous or cancerous cells. In other words, if a woman didn't develop abnormal cells until well into her eighties or nineties, the cancer would not have time to develop and become a problem.

It will be many years before researchers know if they are on the right track: they first need to discover how the immune system deals with pre-malignant cells. Assuming that a wart virus vaccine can be developed, it will take another twenty years to find out if it *works*. With viruses throughout medical history it has always been a case of prevention, or successful intervention, rather than cure.

More money must be put into screening programmes and treatment centres by the government; in particular, more lab technicians must be hired, highly trained and decently paid, and the strictest quality controls observed at testing centres. Colposcopy should move from its exclusive hospital setting and become more GP-based.

Oncologist Tim Oliver wants the importance of genital hygiene stressed through GPs, family planning clinics, obstetric services, STD clinics and sex education classes. If cervical cancer turns out to be a viral cancer as suspected, interleukin 2, when perfected, may be used in a vaccination form to produce a stronger immune reaction. Virus-induced cancers are more likely to be beaten off by a stimulated immune system. We may be only five years away from this form of immunotherapy, and it might be used with the patient's consent on a trial basis when all other treatments have failed. Interferon, a substance that has the ability to inhibit viral growth, may also have a role to play.

Photochemical therapy, or 'light therapy', is the combining of light with certain substances called photo-sensitisers which can selectively destroy tumour cells and leave normal tissue relatively unharmed. Such a photo-sensitiser is porphyrin, which concentrates itself in a tumour. When the tumour is irradiated with ultraviolet light, the porphyrin begins to kill the cancer. There are still some problems with this technique, however, and research is continuing. One drawback is that light therapy is not suitable for large tumours, as light cannot penetrate tissue too deeply – but after a large tumour has been removed by surgery, light therapy can kill any traces of malignant tissue left. At the time of writing it is being used for bladder and rectal cancers, but it is thought that it will eventually work most effectively on cancers of the cervix and vulva.

Last but not least, the future hope for eradicating cervical cancer in its broadest sense must include raising the standard of living/housing for the poor and the elderly, and increasing health and safety standards in certain jobs.

WHAT YOU CAN DO TO HELP YOURSELF

- Get regular smear tests: an early diagnosis is the most important factor.
- Stay faithful to one sexual partner.
- Take care of your and your partner's sexual hygiene.
- If your partner has penile warts, make sure that he gets them treated.
- Stop smoking.
- Use barrier methods of contraception.

If a smear test shows that you have CIN, you might want to see if it will go away by itself without treatment: discuss this with your doctor. Use barrier methods of contraception if you don't already do so; and if you and/or your partner smoke, make a big effort to give up. Your specialist may recommend having an area of abnormal cells removed, especially if you have CIN 2 or CIN 3 – but if you want to wait before having any treatment to see if the condition regresses by itself, or in order to try alternative therapies first, ask your specialist how risky that would be. CIN does not usually develop quickly into cancer – even CIN 3 takes several years to turn malignant – and it may be that all you will need for a while is careful monitoring with frequent smears.

THE COMPLEMENTARY APPROACH

This is the one female cancer with a definite pre-cancer stage which gives you the time you need to try alternative therapies on their own for a time, should you so choose.

Diet

Follow the anti-cancer diet; or you may wish to try one of the other dietary approaches described on pp.186 – 197. Cut down on fats and sugars, as viruses love them.

Vitamins

Take all the vitamins mentioned on pp.197 – 203, but in particular vitamin C, which is known to kill viruses, vitamin A and folic acid, one of the B vitamins, which has been shown in US studies to help women with mild to moderate CIN.

Minerals

Take all the minerals and enzymes mentioned on pp.203-207.

Supplements

Take GLA, bromelain, amino acids and Iscador (see pp.208 – 217).

Herbal Remedies

These are prescribed according to the individual patient's needs, herbs that you may be treated with include Red Clover, Plantain, Cleavers and Mistletoe. All are best taken as teas; the Mistletoe needs to be steeped first in cold water overnight. According to the distinguished herbal consultant Tom Bartram, a herbalist may recommend a vaginal pack to complement treatment for CIN. One such pack consists of Slippery Elm powder mixed with one part Golden Seal in a little water to form a paste. A tampon is saturated with this mixture, and then inserted into the vagina. It is important to note that this is a benign treatment which will not interfere with any orthodox treatment, and which has been found to be helpful in some cases of CIN.

Homoeopathy

Again, treatments given according to individual needs and can sometimes be very effective in the early stages of CIN (See pp.230 – 236).

Other things you might want to try

You could try detoxification (colonic hydrotherapy) though this depends on the degree of spread of CIN (p.221); acupuncture, especially with Chinese herbs (p.239); counselling, relaxation, bio-feedback, breathing exercises (p.244); meditation, visualisation, spiritual healing (p.251).

Some complementary therapists might recommend a caesium douche: this 'caesium' has nothing to do with the radioactive caesium used in internal radiotherapy treatment, but is a harmless metallic salt reputed to kill cancer cells.

7

Endometrial Cancer and Other Rare Women's Cancers

The uterus, also known as the womb, is the organ in which an unborn child develops from a fertilised egg. During pregnancy the uterus expands, but it is normally a 7.5 cm (3 inch)-long hollow organ shaped like a flattened pear. The upper, broader part is the uterus proper; the lower, narrow part which opens into the vagina is the cervix. The terms 'uterine cancer' and 'endometrial cancer' are used interchangeably, as cancer of the uterus almost always begins in the endometrium, or uterine lining. If caught early enough, it is easily curable by surgery.

THE FACTS

- **UK incidence.** In 1984, 3,741 new cases were registered (3 per cent of all cancer registrations).
- **England and Wales five-year survival rate.** From 1981, 70 per cent of patients were alive five years later.
- **UK mortality.** In 1986, 1,050 patients died, with most deaths in the fifty-five to sixty-four age group.

Endometrial cancer rarely strikes before the menopause, and it occurs most often in women aged fifty-five to sixty-nine. It is the commonest gynaecological cancer in the USA. Although there can be different kinds of cancer cells in the endometrium, in 85 per cent of cases the tumour is an adenocarcinoma (a cancer that starts in glandular tissue). It is not a cancer that can be transmitted sexually. It tends to spread through the lymphatic system, rather than the bloodstream; and, like cervical cancer, an endometrial cancer will not become smaller after the menopause – if left untreated, it will simply continue to grow and spread. Its spread is inward, to the lungs, brain and liver. Like breast cancer, it can have a late recurrence. For some reason, older women who get this type of cancer seem to have more virulent tumours.

SYMPTOMS

In pre-menopausal women, who represent only 20 per cent of cases, the symptoms of endometrial cancer are erratic periods or bleeding between periods. For post-menopausal women, symptoms include new bleeding six months after what *appeared* to be the end of the monthly period. This bleeding may start as a watery, blood-streaked discharge which eventually contains more blood. Women should not consider any such extra bleeding to be just a part of 'the change of life': it should always be brought to your GP's attention, so that he/she can find out what is causing it. Eighty-five per cent of this type of bleeding is not due to cancer at all, but to vaginal dryness resulting from menopausal changes. Such dryness can lead to bleeding after intercourse or in connection with an increased risk of candida, or it may become so dry that it bleeds on its own. In pre-menopausal women a benign uterine tumour or fibroid could cause excessive bleeding during periods – in fact, the most common tumours of all are not cancer, but fibroids.

Other symptoms of endometrial cancer for pre- and post-menopausal women include abdominal discomfort or an offensive vaginal discharge.

RISK FACTORS

There may be a slight inherited tendency for this cancer, as it is more common among the relatives of those women who have had endometrial, breast or colon cancer, than among women who have no such disease in their family. Obese women are more at risk, especially after the menopause, as most of our hormones are made in our fatty tissue – and more fatty tissue means more female hormones being produced. Any women on long-term oestrogen drug therapy are also at risk, as the uterus is hormone-sensitive and is stimulated by oestrogen. But any women on hormone replacement therapy (HRT) need not worry, as oestrogen is present with progestogen, which cancels out the oestrogen risk.

Use of the contraceptive pill (according to Kessey's study in Oxford) seems to offer some protection against endometrial cancer, as it does against ovarian cancer, with a degree of protection being extended by duration of use: for up to ten years' pill use, the risk is 20 per cent of that of a non-pill user. But endometrial cancer tends to occur in those women who are infertile, or who have a low number of children, and who may not have taken the pill anyway.

Other risk factors may include hypertension (high blood pressure) and diabetes.

DIAGNOSTIC TESTS

Early diagnosis of endometrial cancer can sometimes be difficult, but if it is caught early, surgery can cure almost all cases. According to David Oram, gynaecological surgeon at the London Hospital, 80 per cent of endometrial cancer is detectable early, or in stage 1 of the disease.

The test for endometrial cancer is scraping away a piece of endometrial lining for examination under a microscope. This is usually done during a dilatation and curettage (D and C) under a general anaesthetic, in a hospital or on an outpatient basis. The cervix is expanded (dilatation) just enough to permit the insertion of a small instrument that removes material from the uterine lining (curettage). This procedure takes only a few minutes, but may be followed by period-type cramps for a day or so, and light bleeding for a week. A woman would know from the results of this test whether or not she had endometrial cancer.

Some treatment centres use a new technology where a jet spray of fluid is injected into the uterus to dislodge cells from the lining for examination.

Other diagnostic tests to check for spread would include chest X-ray, intravenous pyelogram (see p.51 for a description of this), blood tests and abdominal ultrasound.

TREATMENT

Treatment for endometrial cancer consists of surgery or radiotherapy or both, depending on the spread of the disease. Radiotherapy may be used before or after surgery to increase the chance of a cure. In fact, if the cancer cannot be removed surgically, radiotherapy is sometimes the only treatment, and it may be administered externally (see page 96) or internally (see below).

SURGERY

In surgery the womb alone may be taken; if necessary, the Fallopian tubes and ovaries may also be removed. Such a total hysterectomy, however, should be done only if it will effect a total cure. If the cancer is confined to the uterus and has not spread deeply into its muscular wall, it is curable in 90 per cent of cases by removing the uterus and ovaries. If it *has* spread to the muscle wall, internal and external radiotherapy may be given first to reduce the tumour, to be followed by surgery. Around half the patients treated in this way are cured.

See p.35 for a general introduction to surgery and p.91 for more information about hysterectomy.

INTERNAL RADIOTHERAPY

Internal radiotherapy involves inserting radioactive implants resembling tampons into the uterus to fight the cancer from the inside. In the same way as described for cervical cancer (p.97) this technique can narrow the vagina after treatment, and a woman should be told about this possibility beforehand.

Dilators and KY Jelly can be given to help a woman when the vagina narrows.

HORMONE THERAPY/ CHEMOTHERAPY

If the cancer has spread or recurred after treatment, hormone therapy may be used: for instance, progesterone (e.g. Provera), which blocks oestrogen, may be prescribed. There are other hormonal drugs under development which switch off the pituitary sex hormones. In pre-menopausal women, progesterone treatment may sometimes result in a complete regression (disappearance) of the disease. Chemotherapy may also be used.

See pp.39 and 42 for a general introduction to chemotherapy and hormone therapy.

SCREENING

Early screening for endometrial cancer has not taken off in the UK because the various techniques involved are 'intrusive' – that is, they are painful for the 'well' woman and they don't produce specific enough samples for diagnosis. The techniques involve scraping, jet-spraying or sucking out with an instrument a sample of the endometrial lining. The smear test is not useful for endometrial cancer because doctors get a positive smear for only half of those women afflicted: this is due to the fact that abnormal cells shed by the endometrium degenerate before they reach the vagina. So a negative smear could be a false negative.

It is difficult to know the amount of early-stage disease, which is known as 'hyperplasia', in the normal female population. Remarks David Oram, 'It is not acceptable to screen large numbers of asymptomatic women (those showing no symptoms of endometrial cancer), but perhaps we should screen high-risk women: those with obesity, hypertension, diabetes, no

children, or a family history of the disease, as well as those with
symptoms such as abnormal bleeding.'

SURVIVAL

If cancer is confined to the body of the uterus, a woman has a
75 – 80 per cent chance of surviving for at least five years. If the
spread is beyond the uterus, 40 per cent of these women will be
alive five years later. The overall survival rate is 65 – 70 per
cent.

THE ORTHODOX FUTURE FOR
ENDOMETRIAL CANCER

In the opinion of one cancer specialist, this cancer may turn out
to be a sexually acquired virus in the same way as cervical
cancer is thought to be. Future treatment may involve dis-
covering new female hormones and anti-hormones. There may
even be a pill one day to protect against endometrial cancer, as
well as the other two hormone-receptive cancers, breast and
ovarian.

At the moment all a woman can do is to take abnormal or
post-menopausal bleeding seriously, especially if she is in her
forties or fifties – don't hang around, but report any such
bleeding to your GP immediately.

OTHER RARE WOMEN'S CANCERS

Cancer can also occur in the outer genitals, such as the vulva –
that is the labia majora (outer lips), labia minora (inner lips)
and the clitoris; cancer can also occur solely in the Fallopian
tubes or in the placenta. Up to forty cases of cancer of the
placenta, or 'choriocarcinoma' are reported in the UK
annually, and it has at least a 90 per cent cure rate. It can occur
as the result of a pregnancy gone wrong, or after a pregnancy,

when a cancer develops on the part of the placenta where it attaches to the uterus, and gets left behind.

All of these cancers are rare, particularly cancer of the Fallopian tubes, which is usually an extension of ovarian cancer. So uncommon are these cancers that it is difficult to get complete statistics on them, but here is what is available:

- **Cancer of the placenta**
  UK incidence. In 1984, twelve cases were reported.
  England and Wales five-year survival rate. From 1981, 92.5 per cent of cases were alive five years later.
  UK mortality. In 1986, five patients died.
- **Cancer of the vulva, unspecified**
  UK incidence. In 1984, 805 cases were reported.
  Great Britain (England, Scotland and Wales) mortality. In 1986, 420 patients died.
- **Cancer of the labia majora**
  UK incidence. In 1984, fifty-three cases were reported.
- **Cancer of the labia minora**
  UK incidence. In 1984, thirteen cases were reported.
- **Cancer of the clitoris**
  UK incidence. In 1984, twenty-three cases were reported.
  Great Britain mortality. In 1986, six patients died.
- **Cancer of the vagina**
  UK incidence. In 1984, 244 cases were reported.
  Great Britain mortality. In 1986, 120 patients died.
- **Cancer of the Fallopian tubes**
  UK incidence. In 1984, forty-two cases were reported.
  Great Britain mortality. In 1986, fifteen patients died.

There have been no five-year survival rates collected for any of the rarer women's cancers except for cancer of the placenta. Northern Ireland's mortality figures are collected differently, and so could not be included in the above. They group their rare women's cancer mortality figures as follows:

- **Cancers of the ovaries, Fallopian tubes, parametrium and uterine adnexia.** In 1986, ninety-one patients died.
- **Malignant neoplasm of other and unspecified female genital organs.** In 1986, eight patients died.

Vaginal cancer

Like placental cancer, which affects only a tiny minority of pregnant women, vaginal cancer is quite rare, because it requires many associated factors coming together to cause it. The higher incidence is among sixty- to seventy-year-old women, and usually occurs in the upper half of the vagina. Direct spread occurs within the vagina walls and may affect the bladder and rectum in the later stages of the disease. It is thought by some doctors that members of the wart virus family (types 16, 18 and 31) may be involved in initiating cancerous changes. Evaluation by colposcopy is necessary for an accurate picture of the site, size and nature of the lesions involved in vaginal cancer.

The symptoms are vaginal bleeding and/or a foul-smelling discharge, and urinary or bowel symptoms may occur. There may also be pain, depending on the size of the lesion and the degree of spread. Radiotherapy, or radiotherapy in combination with surgery, is being used as orthodox treatment. Because this rare form of cancer is not usually discovered until it has reached an advanced stage, with two-thirds of lesions over 2 cm (0.75 inch) diameter, the orthodox five-year survival rate is around 40 per cent.

Cancer of the vulva

Cancer of the vulva, however, although it is still uncommon, is seen more frequently, particularly at the Royal Marsden Hospital in London. Vulva cancer can sometimes be associated with cervical cancer, but it is also a post-menopausal problem for women in their sixties to eighties: more than 70 per cent of patients are aged sixty or over. Obesity and poor hygiene are almost always involved, although a virus, combined with friction and/or a trauma (damage) is thought to be the *cause*. Hypertension (high blood pressure), diabetes and nulliparity (not giving birth to a child capable of survival) are also considered to be possible risk factors. Overweight women should ensure that their outer genitals are kept clean, and exposed frequently to fresh air. Many women with this cancer have a mass or lumps, usually on the labia majora, and many others complain of pruritis (itching of the vulva). However, itching can also be caused by a plain old vaginal infection (e.g. yeast organisms).

Surgery is normally curative: the operation can take the vaginal lips, clitoris and glands from the groin, leaving the vaginal passage intact, but a *small* lesion can have a very acceptable cosmetic outcome. Larger lesions involve the use of radiotherapy and surgery. Unfortunately, many women seek treatment when the cancer is well established and end up with the more extensive surgery – which is another reason not to delay reporting a sore or small growth in the vulval area. Fortunately, vulva cancer is not on the increase.

WHAT YOU CAN DO TO HELP YOURSELF FOR ENDOMETRIAL CANCER

- Stay slim.
- Avoid oestrogen drugs, except when combined with progesterone, as in hormone replacement therapy.
- Take any abnormal bleeding seriously, whether it is post-menopausal bleeding or between periods.

For the other women's cancers

- Avoid obesity.
- Have regular baths or wash the vagina daily, making sure that you wash between the outer and the inner lips where secretions build up – use warm water, but not soap, which can irritate.
- Wear cotton underwear, and stockings instead of tights, so that sweat is not trapped in the genitals and fresh air can circulate freely in that area.

THE COMPLEMENTARY APPROACH TO ENDOMETRIAL CANCER AND THE OTHER WOMEN'S CANCERS

Diet

Follow the anti-cancer diet, or any of the other diets on pp.186–197. Make sure that any meat or poultry you eat is hormone-free.

Vitamins

All of the vitamins mentioned on pp.197–203 should be taken, in particular Vitamin A (in both its forms), as it has been seen in some studies to cause a regression of epithelial cancers. A good source of vitamin A is halibut oil capsules.

Minerals

Make sure that you are not deficient in any of the minerals mentioned on pp.203–205, in particular zinc and magnesium.

Supplements

Try GLA, bromelain, Iscador (pp.208–217).

Herbal remedies

These are made up for the individual patient, but may include Poke Root and Wild Yam (to clean out the lymphatic system); and Wild Violet leaves, which are believed to inhibit cancer spread. These can be taken as teas, tinctures, fluid extracts, tablets, or capsules. Mistletoe, Red Clover, Plantain or Cleavers may be recommended in tea form: use 2 teaspoons of dried herbs to a cup of boiling water, infuse for fifteen minutes and drink three or more times daily. Steep Mistletoe first in cold water overnight. See pp.226–230.

Homoeopathic remedies

These are made up for the individual, but you may be treated with Asterias Rubens (Red Starfish), which is used for uterine fibroids. See p.233.

Other things that you might want to try

Acupuncture, especially with Chinese herbs (see pp.236 – 243); counselling, relaxation, bio-feedback, breathing exercises (see p.244) and meditation, visualisation, and spiritual healing (see pp.250 – 254).

8

Breast Cancer

The breasts are glands formed mainly from fatty tissue, which contain a system of ducts allowing milk to flow from the milk-producing sacs to the nipple, when needed for breast-feeding. Fibrous support bands link the breasts to the chest-wall muscles. The breasts extend to the armpit, or 'axilla' region, where there are lymph nodes which connect up to the lymphatic system.

THE FACTS

- **UK incidence.** In 1984, 24,471 new cases of breast cancer were reported (19 per cent of all cancer registrations).
- **England and Wales five-year survival rate.** From 1981, 62 per cent of cases were alive five years later.
- **UK mortality.** In 1986, 15,245 died (20 per cent of all cancer deaths).

Breast cancer is the most common form of cancer among women in the UK: each year, around 24,500 women are diagnosed as having it, and around 15,000 die from it. Breast cancer accounts for 20 per cent of all female cancer deaths, and 4.5 per cent of total female deaths. Most deaths from breast cancer occur in the fifty-five to sixty-five age group. It is the commonest cancer for women between thirty-five and fifty-five. A woman has roughly a one in twelve chance of contracting this cancer. Six per cent of women in England stand to contract the disease at some stage in their lives – but if this figure is looked at another way, 93 per cent of English women never get it.

Age is an important factor: women aged over forty are more vulnerable. The incident rate rises from 10 per 100,000 in women under thirty to 150 per 100,000 in women aged fifty and 200 per 100,000 in women aged sixty-five.

England and Wales have the highest mortality rate from breast cancer in the world (28.4 deaths per 100,000), followed closely by Scotland and Northern Ireland (27.7 deaths per 100,000). There has been a slight increase in both the national 'incidence' and 'mortality' rates since 1951 in women over forty-four years of age. The reason for this is not known.

On the world scene, here are the countries in the declining order of mortality after Scotland and Northern Ireland: the Netherlands, USA, Iceland, France, Sweden, Finland, Yugoslavia, Venezuela, Mauritius and Japan. Japan's mortality rate is only 5.8 deaths per 100,000.

There are twenty different categories of breast cancer. Women with certain rare ones like 'tubular ductal carcinoma', representing only 10 per cent of breast tumours, have an excellent chance of recovery. The two most common cancers are epithelial (lining) cancers of either the duct or lobule. Breast cancer can occur in men, but it is a hundred times less common than in women.

SYMPTOMS

Cancer arises in the glandular portion of the milk-secreting section of the breast, or the duct system which transports milk to the nipple. Most breast cancers start in the epithelial lining of the ducts. Cancer of the breast is either 'non-invasive', where the malignant cells are confined entirely within the lobular ducts, or 'invasive', where it spreads into the surrounding tissue.

Some breast cancers grow so slowly that before a lump can be felt, they cause a dimpling in the skin of the breast. Other breast cancers grow so fast that before a lump is felt, some of the cells will have travelled via the blood or lymph. The speed at which cells divide shows how aggressive the cancer is. So what symptoms are you looking for? Basically, you are looking for *any* change in your breasts, and these include:

1. Unusual lump or thickening.
2. Unusual change in the size and shape of a breast. Most women have breasts of unequal size and shape – get to know what is normal in appearance and feel for *you*.
3. One breast unusually higher or lower than the other.
4. Puckering or dimpling of the breast skin.
5. Unusual drawing back of the nipple.
6. Skin trouble such as a rash, in or around the nipple.
7. Swelling of the upper arm.
8. Swelling in the armpit or above the breast (enlarged lymph nodes), or veins that appear to have enlarged.
9. Pain, discomfort or a tingling feeling not felt before, and not confined to the time just before or just after a period.

How to check for symptoms

Breast self-examination (BSE) (see p.121), is the way you go about checking for symptoms on a monthly basis. It is best to examine your breasts a few days after your period if you are still menstruating, or on the same day every month if you have passed the menopause. This way, you won't confuse pre-menstrual, lumpy breasts with any other symptoms.

KNOWING THE DIFFERENCE BETWEEN A CYST, A FIBROADENOMA AND A CANCER LUMP

The reason why you musn't do BSE just *before* a period, is that you may be confused by the normal lumps and bumps that are caused by hormonal influences on the breast ducts.

Cysts

For instance, tiny amounts of fluid from the milk-producing glands can be retained in tiny sacs or 'cysts', which can be tender and painful. Cysts are most commonly found in women in their thirties and forties; they can grow quickly, but they can disappear just as quickly when the period finishes. Very rarely a cancer can mingle with a cyst, so a cyst should never be ignored. Recurring cysts can be drained on an outpatient basis.

Fibroadenomas

The other common pre-menstrual lump found in the breast is a small fibrous lump of glandular tissue called a 'fibroadenoma'. This is also known as a 'breast mouse', as it seems to move around in the breast and can disappear from cycle to cycle. Fibroadenomas are mostly seen in the under-twenty-five age group. If this type of lump persists in a woman over the age of twenty-five, her doctor will probably recommend its removal to be on the safe side, as just occasionally a cancer can mimic a fibroadenoma.

However, it is important to realise that nine out of ten breast lumps are not cancer at all, but a cyst or a fibroadenoma. But remember that any lump which does not change its size with the monthly cycle may not be harmless.

Performing breast self-examination

Although it is best to learn BSE from someone like a nurse who has been trained in the technique, here is a description to help you. Remember to keep in mind the ten symptoms of breast cancer (see above) while you are doing it.

1. Stand before a mirror, undressed to the waist, with your arms at your sides. Look carefully at your breasts, turning from side to side; look underneath them as well.
2. Raise your arms above your head and examine the upper part of the breast that leads to the armpit.
3. Lower and raise your arms again, looking at your nipples – have they each moved upwards the same distance?
4. With hands on your hips, press inwards until your chest muscles tighten, looking for any skin dimpling.
5. Lean forward and examine each breast in turn: is there any puckering, or unusual change in outline?

Do the next three steps either lying down or in the bath, where soapy fingers will make it easier:

6. First examine your left breast with the right hand, feeling with the *flat pads* of the middle three fingers. Using your fingertips can be confusing, particularly if you tend to have glandular breasts. Now press towards the chest wall, using firm but gentle pressure.

    You can mentally divide the breast into quarters, halves, three horizontal sections or a continuous spiral – whichever appeals – as long as you systematically cover the whole breast, the armpit and the top of the collarbone. For pendulous breasts, it might be easier to support the breast with one hand and place the other hand on top to make a sandwich; then roll the breast between the two hands to check for abnormalities.

7. Gently slide your hand over your left nipple and gently squeeze it between thumb and forefinger, looking for any discharge, puckering or retraction.

8. Now repeat steps 6 and 7 on your right breast, using your left hand.

If you do find what appears to be a lump, mark it with a felt-tip pen and see your GP right away. Many women delay seeing their GP after a lump is discovered, out of fear of the diagnosis: but delaying through fear could prevent something potentially serious from being nipped in the bud! And don't forget that nine out of ten lumps are *not* cancer. Pain in the breast is seldom a sign of cancer, but it may signify something else requiring attention.

If you are pregnant, it won't be so easy to do BSE, as your breasts will be going through many normal hormonal changes, so take advice from your doctor. Usually your breasts will be examined for you in the antenatal clinic.

BSE should be carried out monthly by women aged twenty and over. At the age of forty a woman should be going annually to her GP for a clinical examination, and annual mammography should begin at age fifty (see p.153 for more information on mammography). Even when you have annual mammography, you should continue with BSE, as it is not wise to rely on an X-ray alone to discover any lumps.

Some doctors are sceptical about the use of BSE, saying that some cancers have already spread by the time they can be felt.

This is true, but only for a small number of breast cancers. It is not a strong enough reason to take away one of the few positive ways that a woman has of helping herself against breast cancer. And the sceptic's point can be turned on its head: some specialists say that *because* some breast cancers spread so quickly, an annual breast examination by a doctor is not enough, and that women must make regular self-checks for this reason. Women *should* continue to monitor their own bodies: no one can know your breasts as well as you do.

At the time of writing a major trial is taking place in Leningrad to discover whether BSE is important in saving or prolonging life, and the results are awaited with interest. If they are positive, sceptical doctors may once again encourage women to perform BSE.

If you would like to be shown how to do BSE and you are a UK resident, ask at your local family planning or well woman clinic. Or you can obtain a leaflet on BSE from BACUP, the WNCCC, BUPA, the Health Education Council or one of the other organisations listed on p.276.

RISK FACTORS

No one knows what factor or combination of factors triggers off breast cancer. There is probably no one cause, but a complex interaction between an inherited susceptibility, environment, lifestyle, reproductive history, hormone levels and other circumstances. Certain risk factors that are being investigated include: a history of breast cancer in the family; a history of benign breast disease; women who are childless or who delayed their first pregnancy until the age of thirty – the important factor is the number of menstrual cycles up until pregnancy; a long menstrual history of thirty-five years or more; having another cancer, especially of the uterus, ovary or colon; large doses of ionising radiation, as from repeated chest X-rays; and obesity, especially after the menopause. Further details on risk factors can be obtained from the report *Risk Factors for Breast Cancer* by A. Kalache and M. Vessey (see Bibliography).

The genetic link

Although it is true that breast cancer can appear to cluster in the generations of one family, at the very worst a family history only doubles the risk, accounting for just 10 – 15 per cent of cancer victims.

There are, though, some rare family groups where a susceptibility to breast cancer appears to be transmitted genetically. The responsible gene can be transmitted on the father's as well as the mother's side. It travels alongside another gene called the glutamate pyruvate transaminase (GPT) gene, and it can be recognised in a blood test. Women with this gene have a 50 per cent chance of developing breast cancer by the age of fifty, and an 87 per cent chance by the age of eighty – any of their female relatives without the gene, however, have no increased risk.

Research is being carried out to discover if the catalyst for this gene is a cultural or an environmental factor. Industrial pollution may be way down the list of environmental factors, as heavily industrialised countries like Japan still retain low rates of breast cancer. It *is*, however, known that Japanese women, with their overall low risk, take on the higher risk of countries to which they emigrate, within a generation.

The X-ray risk

Women who received multiple X-ray examinations for TB, and for a breast infection called 'acute postpartum mastitis', have an increased risk of breast cancer. The risk goes up in proportion to the X-ray dose received, whether taken as a series of small doses over time, or as one large dose. In this respect, young women's breasts are more vulnerable: for instance, Japanese women exposed as children to the atomic bomb are more at risk.

Myths about breast cancer

The following do *not* cause breast cancer: a knock or blow, fondling, breast-feeding, sunbeds, topless sunbathing, or an active sex life. And large breasts are not more prone to breast cancer than small breasts!

OTHER RISK FACTORS

Under consideration as risk factors are diet (see below), a woman's hormone profile (see p.126), whether a woman is having hormone replacement therapy (HRT, see p.127) and whether she is taking the contraceptive pill (see p.127).

Diet

The cancer epidemiologists Richard Doll and Richard Peto, who were the first to conclusively link smoking to lung cancer, have linked high fat consumption to breast cancer. To a lesser extent, they have also linked meat-eating to the disease. Dietary fats could serve as a vehicle for those carcinogens that are fat-soluble, or it could be that fats depress the immune system. Also, a high-fat diet can alter hormone levels: fatty tissue can make its own oestrogen, which is why obese women are more at risk from breast cancer than slim ones.

Some research has shown that vegetarian women have a lower incidence of breast cancer, which might be due to lower levels of the hormone prolactin, thought to be brought about by a vegetarian diet. But this theory hasn't yet been tested. What needs to be done is a test comparing women who have changed to vegetarian eating with those who have always been vegetarian. It may be that there are other mitigating factors in the lives of vegetarian women.

Although the evidence that changing your diet will reduce your risk of breast cancer is missing, clinical trials have shown that vitamins C and A have inhibited the formation of cancer. So it certainly wouldn't hurt – and it might even *help* – if women ate more foods containing vitamin A, such as dark green and yellow vegetables, and vitamin C, such as citrus fruit.

Almost anything a woman eats can be detected in fluids secreted within her breast ducts: for instance, nicotine appears in a woman's breast secretions after smoking a cigarette. In fact, smoking increases your risk of getting other cancers by 30 per cent, although it doesn't *specifically* increase your risk of breast cancer.

Another diet link is that a high standard of living, and therefore a high standard of *eating* can cause menstruation to start earlier – and the longer a woman is exposed to her own female hormones (the greater number of periods she has before her first conception), the more vulnerable she is to developing breast cancer.

So, playing the orthodox statistics game, women who were fourteen years old and over at the time of their first period have a 20 per cent less chance of developing breast cancer than women who started younger than twelve; women who are fifty-five and older at the start of their menopause have twice the risk of breast cancer as women starting the menopause under fifty; and women who gave birth before the age of eighteen have one-quarter the chance of developing the disease as women who had their first child at the age of thirty. And sticking with the statistics, having a baby after thirty seems to confer a greater risk than not having a child at all!

A woman's hormone profile

Breast cancer is a hormone-dependent cancer. According to one medical view, breast cancer in pre-menopausal women is related to ovarian oestrogens, and in post-menopausal women it is influenced by the conversion of adrenal hormones into oestrogen in the fatty tissue of the body, and is thus related to obesity.

Peter Trott, a cytopathologist says: 'If you removed the ovaries in women before ovulation started, you would cut out breast cancer just like that – the bottom line for breast cancer is too much freely floating oestrogen.' Dr Trott is of course being purposely facetious to make a point, ovaries are *not* taken out to protect against breast cancer, as there are anti-oestrogen tablets which can temporarily stop oestrogen-type hormones from acting.

In 1961 a long-term study of 13,000 healthy women in relation to breast cancer was started on the island of Guernsey by two doctors, Dr Mick Bulbrook of the Imperial Cancer Research Fund (ICRF) laboratories and Mr John Hayward, head of the ICRF Breast Cancer Unit at Guy's Hospital in London. The idea was to track down any pre-disposing factors towards breast cancer.

Although the study is ongoing, two early results link a woman's hormone profile with breast cancer. They are:

1. Women at a higher risk of breast cancer showed lower amounts of certain hormones in their urine up to ten years before diagnosis.
2. Post-menopausal women who have higher levels of oestrogens (more specifically, oestradiol) appear to have about twice the normal risk of developing breast cancer.

The results are interpreted as meaning that hormone variations promote, but don't actually *cause*, breast cancer. More research is needed, because the excess female hormones found in some women may have a positive role to play in another direction, such as protection against osteoporosis and heart disease.

Hormone replacement therapy

Although women who have taken synthetic doses of oestrogen to counteract the effect of the menopause in a singe large dose or over a long period of time may be at risk from breast cancer, the risk of hormone replacement therapy (HRT), which balances oestrogen with progestogen, is more debatable. Medical evidence suggests that HRT taken for longer than ten years increases the risk of breast cancer; but the majority of doctors, including Professor Baum (Professor of Surgery at King's College Hospital and one of the country's leading breast cancer specialists), feel strongly that the benefits of HRT far outweigh the risks, and that HRT is a valuable and safe aid in lessening menopausal symptoms, while also offering protection against osteoporosis and heart disease.

If you are suffering menopausal symptoms and your doctor refuses to give you HRT for reasons connected to your breasts, ask him/her to refer you to a menopause clinic. (A list of such clinics is available from Women's Health Concern – see the list of addresses, p.290.)

The contraceptive pill

More controversial is the link between the birth control pill and breast cancer. Every other day there seem to be new research findings announced that either implicate or exonerate the pill. The confusion is made worse by the fact that testing is done on animals, which cannot adequately predict the cancer risks and benefits in people.

At the time of writing there are two ongoing long-term trials in the UK regarding the pill: one is the Royal College of General Practitioners' (RCGP's) Oral Contraceptive Study, and the other is being run by Martin Vessey and co-workers in Oxford. Neither study has made a clear link between breast cancer and the pill. In fact, Vessey's study (in line with the majority of the thirty studies done so far on the pill and breast cancer) indicates that women from their mid-twenties and older are at no increased risk of breast cancer, even with long-term use of up to twenty years. Where there is still an area of controversy, however, and where the information is still being collected, is in young users (early teens to early twenties), especially those who develop breast cancer early (in other words, has the pill brought forward something that would have developed in those young users *later* in life?). Young users are still a new phenomenon, and they haven't lived long enough for the data to reveal whether they are a group 'at risk' from oral contraceptives – it will be some years before we know for sure.

Although it will be another twenty years before all the data is in from these two studies, the only conclusion to be reached so far is that hormones, in the pill or otherwise, are only likely to encourage cancer rather than initiate it. It must also be remembered that women now take very much lower-dose contraceptive pills than those studied in earlier trials, so that the risks attached to those early years may no longer be relevant. But the most important results of the pill studies relate to ovarian and endometrial cancers: all studies have shown a reduced risk, globally, to 50 per cent of that of a non-pill user, and in some cases, where the pill has been taken for ten years a reduced risk to 20 per cent of that of a non-pill user (see Chapters 5 and 6).

At the moment, the benefits of taking oral contraception seem far to outweigh the hazards. Dr Tim Oliver remarks that the overall evidence is so uncertain that the risk itself, if there is any, is so small as to be insignificant, particularly when the protection against ovarian cancer (and endometrial cancer) from the pill is so clear-cut. Other benefits from the pill include the best contraception protection available, and a release from painful periods; breast fibroadenomas (see p.121) are also less common in women on the pill.

Some doctors believe that the pill might even have a role to play in breast cancer *prevention*, as the synthetic progestogen used in the pill actually inhibits the growth of cancer cells. The 'combined' pill is best, because it also protects a woman from endometrial cancer. For a woman who has had breast cancer, it may even be best for her ovaries to be suppressed by the pill, in order to cut down on the amount of oestrogen floating around in her body.

Stress

Stress is another controversial factor: does it or does it not either contribute to the start of breast cancer or cause a relapse? Some orthodox doctors don't believe that stress is even a co-factor, and that to reduce stress as a complementary therapy for breast cancer has no effect.

Some studies have purported to show that breast cancer has relapsed (regrown) *after* a period of stress. A study undertaken at Guy's Hospital in 1989 showed an association between severe 'life stressors' and a recurrence of operable breast cancer. Whether overall survival from breast cancer is altered by severe stress is not yet known. *How* stress triggers a breast cancer relapse is not yet known but it has been suggested that the neuro-endocrine system and the immune system may play a role. Further studies need to be done on how a woman *copes* with severe stress, and the social support that she gets, as these could be mitigating factors as well. The results are far from proving that stress itself could help to cause the original cancer, and such a study would be very difficult to do.

Another study at King's College Hospital looked at the personality of women with breast cancer and found that the majority of patients suppressed anger, which led to producing stress hormones which could promote cancer growth. But the study is flawed, because it took place *after* the fact: we don't know if the patients repressed their feelings before the discovery of cancer, which would be much more significant. It may be that the *handling* of the stress itself is the most important thing, but as this is an impossible thing to measure, it may have to remain just a theory.

SUMMING UP THE RISKS

At the moment only a woman's age is strongly linked with breast cancer; all the other risk factors are low down on the list, and cannot be used as predictors for the disease. In fact, one US study found that risk factors can explain disease in only about one-quarter of breast cancer patients. Risk factors don't mean that a woman is certain, or even likely, to develop breast cancer. She may be at statistically a greater risk than her neighbour, but her *personal* risk may still be relatively low. Because little is known about the causes of breast cancer, a 'high risk' factor means only a 1 per cent increase in risk.

DIAGNOSTIC TESTS

When a lump or other breast abnormality is discovered, the next step is a series of hospital tests. After the hospital doctor examines the breast and checks for enlarged lymph nodes under the arms and at the base of the neck, a chest X-ray and a blood test will be done to check your general health. This is followed by a **mammography**, a special X-ray of the breasts.

If the lump has fluid in it, **needle aspiration** will be used to draw some fluid off to confirm the diagnosis. If the lump is a cyst, it will disappear at this stage. It is a quick procedure, and can be done in the outpatients' clinic.

If the lump is solid, a **needle biopsy** will be performed: after anaesthetising the area around the lump, a slightly larger needle than that used for aspiration will draw off a small piece of the lump for examination. A negative needle biopsy does not necessarily mean 'all clear', as further investigation by surgical biopsy may be necessary. The doctor may want to remove the whole lump under a general anaesthetic: this is called an **excision biopsy** and may require an overnight stay in hospital.

If cancer is confirmed, further tests may be performed to check whether the cancer has spread. These tests include:

1. **A bone scan.** This is where a slightly radioactive substance is injected into a vein in the arm. Radioactivity will collect

in any areas of the bone where there is abnormal activity, and a scanner will pick this up.

2. **Liver ultrasound scan.** Sound waves and a computer are used to make a picture of the liver, in the same way that a pregnancy is scanned. The procedure is quick and painless, and can measure the size and position of any tumour on or near the liver.

3. **Liver isotope scan.** The liver is also checked in this test. It is similar to a bone scan, in that a low dose of a radioactive substance is injected into a vein. The liver scan is taken twenty minutes later, and any abnormal area will be detected. It is a harmless procedure; the test results take a few weeks to come back.

Other tests that may be used include **xerography**, which is a special X-ray using a different film from the usual X-ray and which outlines the structures of the breast; **thermography**, which is a photograph of the breasts showing areas of increased heat; and **nuclear magnetic resonance**, which are coloured pictures of different body parts using magnetic fields instead of X-rays.

TREATMENTS FOR BREAST CANCER

About 35 per cent of breast cancer patients are 'cured' by orthodox methods, but of that 35 per cent a great number would have lived a long time without any treatment at all: as many as 10 per cent of breast cancers will grow so slowly that a woman dies of something else before she dies of breast cancer.

Orthodox treatment for breast cancer always starts with some form of surgery, followed by radiotherapy, chemotherapy or hormone therapy, or a combination of these. The type of treatment that a patient has will take into account her age, general health, type and size of tumour, its cell type and degree of spread, as well as a patient's preference and a consideration of her personal circumstances. Your hospital doctor will discuss with you the most appropriate surgery for your type of cancer. Discussions are a two-way street (see p.13), so discuss any surgery options carefully, and get all your questions thoroughly answered.

In fact, before any treatment, discuss your feelings with friends and relatives whose judgement you respect, and talk with other women who have been treated for breast cancer. Get all the information that you can from the cancer organisations too (see pp.276 – 279). All of this will help you to make the right decision about your treatment. Only rarely do you need to be rushed into hospital as soon as cancer is diagnosed, so you should have time to explore all the available options. And remember that no surgery can take place without your consent.

SURGERY

Fortunately, the surgical trend is now moving away from mastectomy as being the main option. Many women will be able to have more conservative surgery (see p.35 for a general introduction to surgery), which involves just removal of the lump, followed by radiotherapy. Studies are showing that long-term survival is the same for mastectomy patients as it is for those having the more conservative approach. For women with small invasive lesions of 4 cm (1.5 inches) or less, or with 'in situ' lesions that have stayed in one place, surgery alone may be enough. There are trials currently taking place in the USA and Europe to determine this.

For some types of breast cancer, particularly the fast-growing aggressive ones, mastectomy will be the safest solution. But there is no point in having a mastectomy after the cancer has spread! This is akin to closing the barn door after the horse has bolted. Breast removal can only be justified if it will cure a cancer; or if it prevents the cancer (as in certain types of the disease) from becoming a bleeding, smelly, ulcerated wound on the chest wall, which may be very much worse to bear than a clean mastectomy scar.

If an excision biopsy reveals that a lump is cancerous, there is no need for a surgeon to carry on with further surgery in the same operation. This is the 'frozen section' technique, where a thin slice of the lump is rushed to the laboratory for examination by a pathologist while the woman is still under the anaesthetic – if the slice proves to be malignant, the surgeon carries on with a mastectomy, combining two operations in one.

There is really no need for this, as there is no evidence that cancer spreads between the time of a lump biopsy and that of a second operation. A delay between operations gives the patient time to consider her treatment options, to seek a second opinion if she wants it, to have additional tests to discover the extent of the disease, or to prepare herself emotionally and practically if she decides that it is in her best interests to have further surgery. Fortunately, the frozen section technique is being used less and less.

SURGICAL PROCEDURES

The surgical variations for breast cancer are as follows, and the choice depends on how far the cancer has spread:

Lumpectomy

Lumpectomy is also known as 'Tylectomy'. It is the removal of the affected part of the breast and a few armpit lymph nodes for testing. It is usually followed by radiotherapy and the cosmetic result is good. The advantage is that the breast is not removed; the disadvantage is that there is a greater risk of local recurrence within the retained portion of breast.

Case Study – LUMPECTOMY
In June 1989, when Janet Sadler was forty-seven, a dimple appeared in her breast and she thought she was losing her shape as a result of ageing. Three months later the dimple became a 'funny, lumpy thing' which was painful and Janet experienced pain in her arm, shoulder, back and hips. Her GP sent her to a specialist.

After observing the lump for a seven-week period, the specialist decided to remove it and a few lymph nodes to keep Janet from worrying. A bone scan and blood test were clear. The lump turned out to be cancerous and there were traces of cancer in the lymph nodes, but the specialist was optimistic that he had got it all. When Janet came round from the anaesthetic, she discovered a cut from her nipple to under her arm, with twenty stitches which were taken out a week later. 'It was sore but not too painful,' Janet says. Her worst problem was moving around in bed without disturbing the wound drain. Janet was in hospital only for a weekend. Her lumpectomy was followed by preventative radiotherapy and tamoxifen (see pp.139 and 144), and her first check-up was at six months after treatment. The lumpectomy has left her a bit 'lop-sided' but she says that as she is big-busted, it's hardly noticeable. Five months after her operation her scar was a silver line that was beginning to fade, although she still felt some numbness under the affected arm and she became tired easily.

Partial mastectomy (segmentectomy)

In this operation, a variation on lumpectomy, a quarter of the breast is removed, including the tumour and a wedge of normal tissue surrounding it. Some lymph nodes may be taken. Partial mastectomy is performed in less than 10 per cent of cases. The advantage is that most of the breast tissue is preserved, which is good news for big-breasted women, and there is little chance of loss of muscle strength in the affected arm or of arm swelling. The disadvantage is that cancer may exist in the remaining tissue unless it is treated with radiotherapy; and small-breasted women may be left with a flattened breast.

Case Study – PARTIAL MASTECTOMY OR SEGMENTECTOMY

At the age of thirty-five Pam Iveson found a pea-sized lump in her right breast when in the bath. Her mother had died of bowel cancer six months before. The specialist took out cells from her lump under a local anaesthetic as he thought it would be a cyst, but further examination in a laboratory revealed the cells to be 'dodgy'. Her bone scan showed nothing suspicious. At this point, the surgeon explained that he would like to do a segmentectomy, and asked her to bring in a bra so that he could measure how to hide the scar line under it. Basically, a diamond-shaped piece of flesh and two lymph nodes were removed, and a French pleat was made, consisting of a fine line of stitches, an overlap of skin, and then another fine line of stitches.

Pam says that she was uncomfortable while the stitches were in, but afterwards the breast skin lay flatter without bubbling, and there is only a thin line scar which is hidden by her bra. Her breast is noticeably smaller now, but she doesn't need a prosthesis (artificial breast).

Physically it took her a few weeks to recover, but the odd twinges have continued 'for ages' and her affected arm can't do as much as before: she can't scratch her back with her right arm, for instance, because the chest skin is tighter now. She also had preventative radiotherapy after her surgery (see p.139). Pam now avoids tight clothing and prefers 'bat-wing' sleeves. Emotionally she finds that she's not quite over the experience and that occasionally it 'creeps up' on her.

Simple mastectomy

This is where the affected breast alone is removed. Breast reconstruction may be possible. The advantage is that the chest wall muscle is not removed, arm strength is not reduced, and there is less swelling of the arm as the lymph nodes are left intact. The disadvantage of losing a breast is obvious.

Case Study – SIMPLE MASTECTOMY
In 1982, at the age of forty-three, Jo Stackhouse found a lump in her breast while performing BSE. Although she had a history of lumpy, sore breasts (chronic mastitis), Jo reported her lump straight away to her doctor. A needle biopsy was unable to draw much fluid, and so a biopsy was performed under anaesthetic. The lab results confirmed a malignant tumour hiding under a mastitis lump and the specialist recommended a simple mastectomy. Wanting to get it over with, Jo returned to the operating theatre two days later. She woke up to discover a neat line of thirty-two stitches (nowadays these would be clips). She remarks, 'I wasn't in terrible pain: there was just this pressure in the chest area, and my arm was restricted for a while.' She immediately showed her scar to her husband, and over the months that followed, they watched it heal together.

Because she had found the lump so early, Jo did not need follow-up radiotherapy or hormone treatment and she was back at work eight weeks after the operation. Eight years later her affected arm sometimes aches, especially when she's tired. Jo did feel unfeminine for a while, but her husband was so loving and reassuring that she soon got over the emotional hurt, although she sometimes misses her breast, particularly when on the beach. She now feels fantastic and lucky to be alive.

Eighteen months after her operation, Jo helped to start the Walsall Mastectomy & Breast Cancer Self-Help Group for Women (and

*their families) in her area who experience breast cancer. Her husband
counsels husbands and boyfriends (see the case study on p. 152). Her
experience was a turning point for both of them.*

Modified radical mastectomy

This removes the breast, underarm lymph nodes, and the lining
over the chest muscles. Sometimes the smaller of the two chest
muscles is removed. The advantage is that you may keep your
chest muscles and the muscle strength in the affected arm, arm
swelling is less likely, and it leaves a better appearance than
radical mastectomy; and the survival rate for this operation is
the same as that for a radical mastectomy if it is done early
enough. The disadvantage of losing the breast is again obvious,
and there may be arm swelling.

Case Study – MODIFIED RADICAL MASTECTOMY

*Margaret Harvey was forty-five when she found a lump to the right
of her sternum, which felt like a bit of gristle on her rib. Her doctor
was unconcerned and so didn't offer her a mammogram, and did
nothing further about it for thirteen months. Suddenly feeling a sense
of urgency, she went to a local hospital clinic where her lump was
removed under a local anaesthetic. The lump turned out to be a
'lympoma' (fatty tissue) with a bit of cancer attached – she was told
that her right breast would have to be removed.*

*Margaret had a good cry before the operation, but found after-
wards that there was more soreness and numbness than pain. She
was bruised from her collarbone down to her diaphragm, but the
bruises faded after a few days. After six weeks she was given a proper
prosthesis to wear. Margaret felt some bony rib pain for some months
afterwards, as well as electric sensations like nerves jumping, and
she thought that she had cancer secondaries. However, her oncologist
and other mastectomy patients reassured her that this was part of the
normal healing process.*

*Six years later, some parts of her chest leading into the armpit are
still numb to the touch, but this is also normal. She believes that this
is a small price to pay as her cancer has not recurred. Margaret also
experienced chemotherapy and radiotherapy (see pp. 139 and 141).*

Radical mastectomy

In this operation the breast, armpit glands, chest muscles and some fat and skin are removed. Breast reconstruction is sometimes possible (see p.148). The advantage is that the cancer can be completely removed, if it has not spread beyond the breast or nearby tissue. The disadvantage is that it leaves behind a long scar and a hollow chest area, may cause some loss of arm muscle power and may create restricted shoulder motion. This operation is now uncommon.

Case Study – RADICAL MASTECTOMY
In 1972 when Susan Gurney was thirty-six, a benign lump was removed from her left breast. Three years later another lump was removed from the same breast, but this time the biopsy revealed something suspicious. Susan sensed that she was headed for a radical mastectomy but was stoical about it, as she realised the breast had always been a source of trouble. She was well strapped when she came round from the surgery, but after three days the dressing came off and a light pad was placed over the wound. On the third day after the surgery she felt weepy, mostly, she says, because she felt uncomfortable.

She was given exercises to do in the hospital and at home, but it was six weeks before she could lift her arms above her head. Ten days after her hospital discharge Susan was fitted with a prosthesis, and she stresses the importance of getting a well-fitting bra. She experienced very slight lymphodoema (accumulation of lymph) in her left arm and was told not to do any lifting for a while. Her arm recovered over a four-month period. From time to time over the six months that it took Susan to get fully back to normal, she felt a 'tightening sensation' around her chest, and numbness down the back of her arm. Even now, at the age of fifty-four, there are still spots where it's numb. At first her post-operation check-ups were every three months and then every six months, but now they are once a year.

Always ask your surgeon if it is possible to have a lumpectomy or a segmentectomy, followed by radiotherapy. Mastectomy should always be the last choice, although it is interesting to note that in a study done in Newcastle General Hospital between 1979 and 1987, fifty-four out of 153 breast cancer patients chose conservative treatment, and ninety-nine chose mastectomy. The reasons for this choice were a desire for rapid results; employment or domestic arrangements; or a fear that a future mastectomy might have to be done anyway, even though the study was biased towards the conservative therapy. The Cancer Research Campaign has also funded studies which reveal that one-third of women involved in their trials opted for mastectomy when given a genuine choice.

Newcastle General did stop offering a choice of conservative treatment to patients with lobular cancer, as the risk of recurrence is three times higher than that of ductal cancers. They also emphasised mastectomy for those breast cancers like 'in situ' lesions (a cancer that stays in the place where it started), which have a high cure rate with this operation. During the follow-up, no advantages to conservative treatment or mastectomy were noticed in terms of recurrence or survival.

Reducing the hormone prolactin before surgery

Prolactin is a hormone secreted in women by the pituitary gland. It is connected with lactation (milk production) and is produced in larger than usual amounts by women suffering any kind of stress, including facing breast cancer surgery. Prolactin can stimulate breast cancer cells to multiply if they are shed from the tumour at the time of surgery.

In 1988 a team led by the Imperial Cancer Research Fund's clinical oncology unit at Guy's Hospital began trials to block prolactin production for a period of time before and after surgery, by giving a drug called bromocriptine. The results of the trial, involving thirty-eight women, showed lower levels of prolactin in the bromocriptine group than in the placebo group; and when the breast tumours removed were examined, far fewer multiplying cells were found in the women taking the drug. Further research is taking place into what may be a new way to reduce the risk of breast cancer recurrence. Another bit of good news is that the drug has no side effects.

RADIOTHERAPY

It may be mutually agreed between patient and specialist that radiotherapy (see p.36 for a general introduction) is the best treatment after surgery. Before radiotherapy, some or all of the underarm lymph nodes are usually removed and examined in the lab to help the oncologist to 'stage'the disease. The stages are these:

Stage 0, a carcinoma 'in situ'.
Stage 1, a small mobile tumour less than 2 cm (0.75 inch) across which is confined to the breast, with no lymph node involvement and no known spread.
Stage 2, the same as stage 1 only with some lymph nodes involved; or a larger tumour – 2–5 cm (0.75–2 inches) – with or without nodes involved. Again, there is no known spread. Up to this point it might be possible to avoid a mastectomy.
Stage 3, a 'locally advanced' tumour which may be attached to the chest wall, with some nodes involved, but no known distant spread.
Stage 4, distant spread, or metastasis, is present.

Radiotherapy treatment is aimed at the breast and at those nearby areas which still contain some lymph nodes, such as under the arm, above the collar bone and along the breastbone. About five weeks after surgery, most women will receive a concentrated booster dose of radiation to the area where the breast lump was located. This is done either through external radiotherapy or internally with an implant of radioactive material.
External radiotherapy side effects include an irritation of the skin affected, nausea and fatigue, but these gradually disappear when the treatment finishes. There may be some small broken blood vessels left on the skin where treatment took place.

Case Studies – EXTERNAL RADIOTHERAPY
Janet Sadler had radiotherapy two months after her lumpectomy, five days a week for four weeks. She felt unwell straight away, and was sick, but she was given tablets which helped her most of the time. She was put on two different radiotherapy machines each day of her

treatment, which covered her lymph nodes up to her neck and also her back. Her skin was very red and sore up to ten days after treatment, and she peeled badly.

Pam Iveson was given radiotherapy treatment a month after her segmentectomy. She had twenty-three treatments in all, with four sites treated. For four weeks during treatment time she was on a linear acceleration machine which doesn't touch the skin and for three weeks she was on a cobalt machine which does touch the skin, and so requires lead shielding. Pam developed a bad sunburn and sickness (medication helped to contain the nausea) and has permanently lost the hair under her right arm and on the back of her neck, and the skin pores in both places are now 'waxy-looking'. Her advice for coping with such treatment is to rest and sleep it off, as it also made her feel very tired. It took a few weeks after treatment ended for all her symptoms to disappear and about nine months to get her energy levels back.

Margaret Harvey had radiotherapy after chemotherapy treatment over a six-week period, with five days on and two days off. She experienced no side effects, not even fatigue, but she did develop an infection (cellulitis) around the wound which required antibiotics to clear it up.

Elizabeth Wood, who had a radical mastectomy on her right breast in early 1960 and simple mastectomy on her left breast in 1989, found herself facing radiotherapy again at the age of eighty-six. She had twenty-two sessions in three different positions, plus three booster sessions. She felt sick but could still eat plain things like cereal and bread and butter. She also developed a bad sunburn, which lasted for three weeks. ' I couldn't bear to clamp my arms to my sides,' she says. She healed very well, however, and the only lasting effect was that the lymph nodes on her left side stopped functioning as a result of the radiotherapy.

Internal radiotherapy

For internal radiotherapy treatment, wires of irridium are planted in the affected breast under a local or a general anaesthetic, to give an extra dose of radiation to the area around the tumour. This can now be done immediately after conservative surgery, under the same anaesthetic.

First, thin plastic tubes are threaded through the breast tissue where the original lump was removed: the number and the location of the tubes depends on the size and position of the original tumour. Then, in the privacy of your own hospital room, radioactive seeds, usually of irridium, are inserted into the tubes. The wires usually remain in place for three to four days. During this time, you are a small risk to those coming into contact with you because of the radioactivity being emitted, and so visiting is restricted. The radioactivity disappears, however, when the wires have been removed, which is much like having stitches out. The whole procedure is uncomfortable, but not painful, and there is no scar afterwards.

A new approach leaves the implants in place for only forty-eight hours and then the patient is given external radiotherapy on an outpatient basis. Doctors are now trying to discover if an increased dose of radiotherapy in the implant might avoid the need for external radiotherapy.

After internal radiotherapy, changes in the breast may continue for six to twelve months. They include a sunburn that becomes a tan, enlarged pores, an increase or decrease in skin sensitivity, and breasts that feel firmer or larger. The firmness or 'largeness' is due to a build-up of fluid or fibrous tissue. If a year after treatment you experience any changes in the size, shape, appearance or texture of your breasts, report these to your doctor at once.

CHEMOTHERAPY

The use of aggresive chemotherapy in breast cancer is gradually receding in many countries, but this form of treatment may be used in addition to radiotherapy when cancer has also been found in the underarm lymph nodes, as it can reach areas of the body where cancer cells may be hiding. (See p.39 for a general introduction to chemotherapy.)

It is also given after surgery or radiotherapy to women at risk of their cancer recurring – even if there is no sign of the cancer present. Used in this way, it is known as 'adjuvant chemotherapy', and it has delayed or prevented the recurrence of breast cancer in patients whose cancer had reached one or more of the lymph nodes removed during the initial surgery. Chemotherapy may also be used later for secondary tumours.

A combination of cytotoxic drugs is best for breast cancer: for pre-menopausal women where cancer has spread to the lymph nodes, it has reduced the risk of dying over the next five to perhaps ten years by 30 – 40 per cent. Unfortunately, it is of no value in treating post-menopausal women. The drug combination most frequently used is cyclophosphamide, methotrexate, fluorouracil (CMF). It is now known that six courses of CMF are as effective as and less toxic than twelve courses. There is no evidence to suggest that taking CMF for longer than six months is any more effective.

Research is now looking into whether a two-drug combination is as effective as a many-drug combination. In general, chemotherapy can make a breast cancer patient comfortable, but is may cure only one in ten or twenty. However, between them chemotherapy and radiotherapy have helped 20 per cent of pre-menopausal women. As it is known that continuous infusions of drugs can minimise their toxicity, the future of chemotherapy may involve small pumps that a patient could wear, which would pump smaller amounts of the drugs into her bloodstream over a longer period of time.

The number of courses of a drug prescribed depends on the cancer type and on how well it is responding to the drugs. Treatment is given over a few days, either in the hospital or on an outpatient basis, which is followed by a rest period of a few weeks to allow the body to recover from any side effects. Treatment may continue intermittently for many months. Whereas surgery and radiotherapy treat a localised area, chemotherapy has the advantage of distributing drugs capable of destroying cancer cells throughout the body.

See p.41 for information about the possible side effects of chemotherapy, which are not experienced by all patients apart from tiring more easily and being more prone to infection.

Case Studies – CHEMOTHERAPY

Margaret Harvey had chemotherapy treatment immediately after her surgery for modified radical mastectomy, followed by six weeks of radiotherapy. She was then put back on a course of chemotherapy as a preventative, which consisted of an intravenous injection of three drugs on the first and seventh days of the month for eight months. She also had to take six tablets a day for the first fourteen days of every month. The intravenous treatments made her feel 'hot and ill', and though she didn't vomit, she felt very sick. The worst part of it for her was the hair loss, but she was fitted with a wig as soon as a few bald patches occurred, which saved her further anxiety. She had to miss her eighth treatment because her white blood cell count was too low. Five and a half months after chemo treatment finished her hair had grown again and long enough for her to go without a wig for the first time.

Margaret Brice went on chemotherapy two weeks after a mastectomy as part of the Midland Breast Trials in 1979. It was a new treatment involving six cytotoxic drugs, and one treatment was given every third week for eight sessions. Each treatment took from a Tuesday lunchtime to a Wednesday morning. Sickness affected her from the second treatment onwards, and got progressively worse, although anti-sickness injections helped. Her hair soon began to fall out after the second treatment, so she had her hairdresser cut and style a wig for her. Every Tuesday morning she would eat as much as she could, because she knew that she wouldn't be able to eat for a few days after treatment. By the third treatment she 'didn't know if she could cope', but her doctor gave her a tranquilliser and she went into her fourth treatment feeling calm. She missed one treatment while her iron levels were built up, and then had the full course. The treatment did knock her ovaries out of action, and she experienced hot flushes, dry skin, a dry vagina and mood swings — some of these symptoms lasted as long as two years. Her hair grew back fluffy and fuzzy, and a lighter colour. In 1983 she founded the Walsall Mastectomy & Breast Cancer Self-Help Group with Jo and Brian Stackhouse (see the case study on page 135).

HORMONE THERAPY

Hormone therapy (see p.42 for a general introduction) is used on those cancers whose cells are responsive to hormones. In patients with such cancers the glands that produce hormones (the adrenals, pituitary and the ovaries) were at one time surgically removed, but now hormones can be suppressed by chemicals such as tamoxifen. Sometimes hormone therapy is given immediately after surgery or radiotherapy, or it can be used as 'adjuvant therapy', to help those women thought to be at a risk of recurrence.

In pre-menopausal women a remission in breast cancer can occur if the amount of female hormone in the body is reduced or a male hormone is taken. In post-menopausal women there is a favourable reaction if the hormone balance is changed in *either* direction.

The more oestrogen receptors on your cancer, or if it is a secondary cancer, the longer the time between its discovery and the curing of the primary cancer, the more hormone-receptive it is likely to be. There is more than one way to change your hormone balance, so if the treatment you are on hasn't worked, your doctor can prescribe a different one.

TAMOXIFEN

Tamoxifen is an anti-oestrogen drug which is often given to post-menopausal cancer patients instead of radiotherapy or chemotherapy, and sometimes even instead of surgery when an operation might be risky, as, for example, in the case of an elderly woman. Tamoxifen is as good as radiotherapy in post-menopausal women, especially where there is a small tumour; and in fact this patient group tends to get more hormone dependent cancers. When tamoxifen is given to patients over the age of fifty for two years after their initial treatment, there is both a reduced relapse rate and a reduction in the risk of death – from 30 to 24 per cent – over five years.

Tamoxifen therapy is given to younger patients after radio-therapy and chemotherapy. In patients under fifty, though, there is no convincing evidence of a reduced mortality rate following this therapy, although there is good evidence of a reduced relapse rate.

In early breast cancer, tamoxifen works for both older and younger patients in reducing the death rate when used as the only treatment after surgery. In a study of 1,285 women treated with the drug for two years after a mastectomy for early breast cancer, the death rate at the six-year follow-up was found to have reduced by 34 per cent. Results were independent of age, the number of lymph nodes involved or the tumour's degree of oestrogen receptivity.

Tamoxifen works by blocking the reception of the oestrogen produced in the adrenal glands; the hormone gonadotrophin is used to suppress oestrogen made in the ovaries. But tamoxifen may also inhibit cell growth factors. For women at high risk of developing cancer, the drug can reduce the activity of free oestrogen – that is, oestrogen not bound to other molecules in the system. Even if a patient's tumour is oestrogen- or progesterone-negative, tamoxifen will be used to start with, to avoid having to use chemotherapy.

Tamoxifen has been mentioned as a possible preventative treatment for high-risk women, but before this can happen, the long-term risks of tamoxifen therapy need to be studied. One study indicates that after five years use there is a slightly increased risk of endometrial cancer. We are still a few years aways from a preventative trial.

Case Study – TAMOXIFEN (HORMONE THERAPY)

Janet Sadler was put on hormone therapy in July 1989, a month after her lumpectomy. She was prescribed tamoxifen tablets, one a day, and reckons she will be on them for a long time to come. During the first two or three days of taking the tablets, Janet experienced dizziness and blurred vision, but these symptoms quickly went away and she doesn't know for sure if they were due to the tamoxifen.

Freda Chapman was put on tamoxifen after having a modified radical mastectomy in 1988 at the age of forty-six. Cancer had been found in the lymph nodes so Freda knew that there was no guarantee that the cancer wouldn't come back. Her specialist advised her to 'think positive', and to stay on tamoxifen therapy for the rest of her life. She has had no side effects from it, and when she runs out of tablets she simply obtains more from her GP.

Sometimes the drug aminoglutethimide is used after a relapse following tamoxifen therapy – it, too, can stop the adrenal glands from producing hormones like oestrogen for as long as the drug is taken. Although theoretically it can cause a remission of any cancer sensitive to male and/or female hormones, aminoglutethimide is not as good as tamoxifen and is more toxic. But between the two drugs, 30 per cent of breast cancer patients have experienced one to two years of remission (that is, their cancer has shrunk, though this does not mean that they are cured).

Other hormone drugs used include corticosteroids, which can also produce a remission by temporarily inactivating the adrenal glands; and progesterone, which can help those who develop a secondary cancer of the uterus, as it causes a remission of this secondary cancer in one in three patients.

Although the female hormones seem to have no side effects worth mentioning, the male hormones certainly do, and these include thinning head hair, growth of hair on the chin and upper lip, acne, a deepening of the voice, ankle swelling and sometimes even yellow jaundice. If you are not prepared to put up with such side effects, ask your doctor to try another hormone preparation. For all the benefits of hormone therapy, it must be said that some breast cancers can learn to live without their hormone dependency and so may not respond to treatment.

As with any course of treatment, your progress will be checked regularly, but as time passes your appointments will become less and less frequent. Your GP will be kept informed as to your progress by your hospital doctor.

MASTECTOMY AND AFTER EFFECTS

Eighty per cent of operations now done for breast cancer are not mastectomies, but mastectomy is still considered to be the best treatment for tumours which are multifocal, are over 4 cm (1.5 inches) in diameter, are high in grade, or which are sited behind the areola (the darker-coloured area surrounding the nipple). It may also be the choice of a woman with a smaller tumour to reduce the risk of local recurrence and the need for radiotherapy.

After a mastectomy, your arm on the side treated will feel stiff and you will be given arm exercises to do. Physiotherapy is very important, as moving your arms and shoulders as soon as possible after surgery will help prevent them becoming stiff. Swimming is good too, but you will not be allowed to swim during radiotherapy treatment. (See pp.132 – 138 for more information on mastectomy, and on the emotional effects this operation can have on patients.)

Lymphoedema

If your lymph nodes were removed during breast surgery, this can make the hand and arm nearest your affected breast vulnerable to infection: a small cut, burn or graze may become sore as a result of a flow of lymphatic fluid from other parts of the body. Don't wear tight jewellery or tight sleeves; wear gloves while gardening, washing up or handling dishes of hot food; wear a thimble while sewing; use an electric razor instead of an ordinary one; and treat insect bites or cuts immediately.

If the affected arm swells or feels very sore, you could have lymphoedema (an accumulation of lymph in the tissues). Tell your doctor at once, so that he/she can prescribe the necessary drugs to cure it.

Breast prosthesis

After a mastectomy, you will be given a lightweight foam prosthesis, or artificial breast, to put inside your bra, and it will match your breast in size and shape. You can be fitted for a more permanent prosthesis after six to eight weeks, or two to three weeks after radiotherapy. You don't need a special mastectomy bra; an ordinary sports bra will hold a prosthesis perfectly well. As the prosthesis acts like a natural breast, you can wear any clothes that suit an ordinary bra too. Women who have had a mastectomy are entitled to a refund of the 15 per cent VAT on their clothes – ask the Breastcare and Mastectomy Association (BCMA) for their booklet *Looking Good After Surgery* if you want information about this. The prosthesis will need to be washed and cared for like skin, and you can even swim in it.

There are several types of prosthesis available on the NHS, and you are entitled to a silicone prosthesis every two years. You may want to buy one privately, though, as there is more diversity of choice, and the BCMA can supply you with a list of private stockists throughout the country (see the list of addresses on p.276). The BCMA also has a permanent exhibition of swimwear and underwear at its London headquarters. Wherever you obtain your prosthesis – from a nurse, surgical appliance fitter or the BCMA – make sure that you are happy with it.

It is not well known that you can obtain a *partial* prosthesis, which would be suitable if you had a lumpectomy which had changed the shape of your breast.

However, some women may not want to wear a prosthesis at all, and this is up to them – remember that no one should force you to do anything that you feel uncomfortable doing.

BREAST RECONSTRUCTION

The same applies to breast reconstruction. Any woman who has had a mastectomy should be able to have breast reconstruction, even if the breast skin is thin, or tight, or there is an absence of chest muscles. You may not care for the additional surgery that this entails, and be perfectly happy just to wear a prosthesis, or none at all – but it is important to have a choice.

If you *do* opt for reconstruction, ask you doctor to refer you to a plastic surgeon who has done a lot of these operations and ask him/her exactly what you can expect. For some women, a reconstructed breast contributes to their feeling of wellness and 'wholeness'.

The best results are obtained from using muscle and skin from another part of the body – for instance, the back of the chest wall – and using this tissue together with an implant to build up a naturally contoured breast. A newer technique for breast reconstruction involves putting an expanding silicone implant under the pectoralis major muscle, then injecting saline weekly until it is slightly over-expanded. At that point, the silicone expander is taken out and a silicone prosthesis with a bit of natural droop is put in.

Some surgeons will do a reconstruction straight after a mastectomy; others like to wait three to six months for the mastectomy scar to be well healed. But reconstruction can be performed years after a mastectomy with good results, even on women in their seventies.

To help you to make up your mind, discuss reconstruction

with your friends and family, and talk to other women who have had it done – and women who have decided *not* to have it done. If you know that you want a breast reconstruction before you have your mastectomy, speak to your surgeon prior to any surgery as the position of the mastectomy incision may affect the reconstruction procedure. If your surgeon won't agree to a reconstruction, ask him/her to refer you on for a second opinion: he/she shouldn't object, as he/she will either have his/her opinion confirmed, or both of you will have the benefit of two expert opinions before making a final decision.

An **immediate reconstruction** is simpler as no drainage tube is needed and quite often absorbent stitches can be used – but it makes your hospital stay a bit longer: you could be in for two weeks. A **secondary reconstruction,** which means returning to hospital at some later point, presents a problem only if there has been a great deal of skin loss: the size of the new breast may be greatly restricted. But a **partial restoration,** offering a cleavage, may be possible.

There are several types of implant used, the simplest being of silicone rubber filled with silicone gel. (By the way, there is no evidence that silicone causes cancer.) The implants come in various sizes, and are chosen to match the remaining breast as closely as possible.

Case Study – SECONDARY BREAST RECONSTRUCTION

Brenda Thompson had undergone a modified radical mastectomy on her right breast in May 1984 at the age of forty-one and hadn't given breast reconstruction a thought. A year later, at her check-up, her specialist had said that she was a good candidate for secondary breast reconstruction, and as she had had a small cancer, he had left a little piece of flesh near the cleavage during her surgery to give her a future option. The specialist asked Brenda to wait for two years before having the operation to ensure that there would be no recurrence of the cancer, and in 1986 she decided to go ahead with it.

'It wasn't that I felt disfigured,' she said, 'but dressing and un-dressing constantly reminded me of my loss.' And two reconstruction patients reassured her with their results.

In the operating theatre she remembers seeing what looked like a square of yellow unset jelly: this was the silicone implant. She was under anaesthetic for only an hour and her new breast was only a bit

*sore afterwards, although it was bruised, red and swollen. She could
have had her right nipple reconstructed in the same operation, but as
it would have made the operation much longer she decided not to. She
went home the day after the operation, because everything was fine.
She was given painkillers, but needed only one, and four days after
going home any little pain had disappeared. After seven days her four
stitches were removed, which wasn't painful.*

*It took six months for the bruising to go completely, and within
that time the breast got a bit harder, 'but not rock-hard — six months
is the limit to how hard it will get'. Brenda says that her new breast
'moves with me, and feels a part of me', and she now enjoys wearing
sundresses and bathing suits that she would have avoided before. Her
only problem (a small one) was that the blood circulation took a
month to return in full to the top of her new breast where the skin is
thin. She also had to avoid any heavy lifting for a few months.*

*The new breast was checked after six months and then at yearly
intervals. The specialist checks for any adhesions, but there haven't
been any so far. The reconstruction scar has faded to a silvery line,
which can't be seen anyway. Brenda's husband is very pleased with
the results. 'It was so simple,' she says.*

Nipple/areola reconstruction

It is rare to be able to preserve the original nipple after mastectomy, so if you want a new nipple or areola (the dark area surrounding the nipple), you may well require a second operation
six to twelve months later. The hospital stay can be anything
from a few days to a week. The areola is reconstructed by using
skin from the upper inner thigh or behind the ear, whereas the
nipple is reconstructed from the tissue of the new breast mound,
or by grafting a piece from the remaining nipple. However the
nipple is done, it won't look or feel like a normal one, and you
may prefer a moulded one, which is held on by cream.

Bear in mind also that although the original mastectomy scar
can be improved in appearance, it cannot be eliminated.

Complications with breast reconstruction

There can sometimes be complications with breast reconstruction: in 25 per cent of patients 'capsular contracture'

occurs, where a fibrous capsule forms around the implant. When any foreign body enters under the skin, the body tries to wall it off with fibrous tissue (for example, the fibrous capsule mentioned here). This fibrous tissue is completely benign and is a natural reaction – the body's way of defending itself against what it deems an invasion by a foreign substance. Occasionally the capsule can thicken and cause discomfort, and if the surgeon cannot break the capsule through manipulation, further surgery will be required.

Sometimes a cancer can develop and hide behind an implant, making detection difficult – although the pro-breast reconstruction lobby refutes this. A few cancer cells may also linger if the surgeon is trying to preserve the original nipple, and this procedure must be carefully thought about beforehand and done with care to ensure that all the original breast tissue is removed from behind the nipple. But breast reconstruction itself does not speed up the spread of cancer.

Where to find a surgeon

You can sometimes have breast reconstruction performed on the NHS, and a list of surgeons who are willing to do it is obtainable from the BCMA and the British Medical Association (see the list of addresses on p.276).

COUNSELLING FOR MASTECTOMY

Breast cancer, where it involves mastectomy, is the only one of the four women's cancers to be immediately apparent, if not to the outside world, to a woman's partner and family. A woman who has had a mastectomy will be feeling profoundly sad at the loss not just of a part of her body, but of all it represents: her femininity and part of her sexuality and self-image. There will be a mourning period; there may also be feelings of anger.

How to deal with such a great feeling of loss and make decisions about a prosthesis or reconstruction at the same time can be overwhelming when a woman is feeling vulnerable and unwell. The BCMA runs a nationwide volunteer support programme staffed by women who have been through the mastectomy experience themselves, so they will be able to give you all the emotional support you need, as well as answer your non-medical questions.

A woman's partner may be in a state of shock as well, or not sure how to react. If she makes sure that he is part of any discussion with doctors, nurse-counsellors and other professionals from the start, he should be better able to adjust. This is especially true about discussions concerning the kind of surgery, or about prosthesis *versus* breast reconstruction, so that he will know what to expect.

Case Study – COUNSELLING FOR MEN

When his wife, Jo, told him that she must undergo a mastectomy because of breast cancer, Brian Stackhouse was utterly despondent and could think of only one thing: the possibility that she might die. He had worked as a Samaritan and had known two women who had died of breast cancer.

Jo told her husband and family about the mastectomy when they were all together, and they all had a good cry. Says Brian: 'When one of us has a problem, we all have a problem.' However, Jo's confidence gave Brian more confidence to deal with it, and he kept himself busy thinking of the good times they had had and the good times yet to come. Immediately after the surgery, Jo showed him her scar and he continued to look at it daily with her, watching it heal. He found that he didn't react badly to the scar. When Jo came home from hospital, Brian found himself being over-protective of her and admits he 'treated her like a patient' for longer than necessary. At that time there was no counselling available in the area, except what was given to them by their daughter, who is a nurse. Brian took an active interest in all the breast cancer books that Jo read.

When Jo founded the Walsall Mastectomy & Breast Cancer Self-Help Group, Brian decided to help counsel the boyfriends and husbands. He found the men all asked the same first question: 'Is she going to live?' His answer to this was that there is no real answer; that it depends on the type of breast cancer and how long it's been left. Later, after the surgery, Brian would ask the men how they felt about their partner's altered body image and whether their relationship was the same as before the operation. He found that 80 per cent of the men he counselled who were under thirty-five were exceptionally understanding and were prepared to wait a while until their spouse's sex drive came back. In men over the age of fifty, Brian found that a similar proportion were supportive, but he noted that between the ages of thirty-five and fifty there were some problems with the men's reactions: some of these men didn't know enough about their wife's condition and reacted badly, rejecting her or turning to alcohol or infidelity. Brian considers the age group thirty-five to fifty to be a 'dangerous one' for men involved with women who have breast cancer, even if they are already in a healthy marriage. Some men are unable to talk about their deepest feelings and fears straight away, he says, 'but all of them gain hope by seeing how well Jo is'.

Brian helps the men to find their sense of humour while under immense emotional strain. He notes that more sexual problems result from the cancer if the marriage wasn't strong beforehand, but that the friendship element keeps couples going over the worst hurdles. 'The majority of men and women will learn to accept the woman's altered body image as just another phase in their relationship which can be got through,' he says.

SCREENING WITH MAMMOGRAPHY

There has been much debate over the use of mammography as an early screening device for breast cancer: who should have it, and when. Randomised controlled trials in New York and Sweden and case-control studies in the Netherlands and Italy (see the Glossary, p.262, for explanations of these terms) have finally clarified that regular mammography will cut down the death rate from this cancer by at least one-third to one-half for women over fifty. Screening for women under fifty has not yet proved effective, as younger women have denser breast tissue in which it is more difficult to detect changes. Further research, however, may demonstrate a benefit from lowering the age for routine screening.

From March 1988 health authorities in the UK have begun phasing in the National Breast Screening Programme, which aims to achieve a 30 per cent reduction in mortality among women aged fifty to sixty-four by the end of the century: that is a minimum of 3,000 lives saved a year. A nationwide service should be established by 1990. Women will be screened at three-yearly intervals, although this time interval will be kept under review. Women over sixty-five will be screened on request, while those under the age of fifty with symptoms can be referred to a breast specialist by their GP.

Research shows that screening every two to three years poses no cumulative risk from the age of fifty and over, but that if annual screening is started prior to this age, there is a danger of a woman accumulating too much radiation over her lifetime. The dose of radiation for a single mammogram is a fraction of a rad: a cancer risk equivalent to smoking a third of a cigarette.

Single-view mammography

Screening consists of a 'single-view' mammogram: this is where each breast in turn is compressed against an X-ray plate while the film is being exposed, and it is uncomfortable for a few seconds. The film is processed and read under the supervision of a consultant radiologist.

Screening itself does not reach an absolute verdict on whether cancer is present: it simply sorts out the screened population into 'test postive' and 'test negative'. If the results are normal (that is, 'test negative'), the woman and her GP will be informed and the woman is recalled in three years' time. If the mammogram is abnormal ('test positive'), the woman will be asked to attend an assessment centre for further tests, to discover whether the growth is benign or malignant. Specialist screening teams consist of a radiologist, a doctor who may also be a surgeon, a radiographer, a nurse and a histopathologist. The standard of those who do the screening must be very high, and the government will need to keep a constant watch on this.

False positives

About 70 – 80 per cent of screen-detected cancers have a good prognosis, but screening can come up with some 'false positives': this is when the mammogram shows what *appears* to be a cancerous lump, which a biopsy reveals to be benign. As a result of this screening, some women will be over-treated, with biopsies that will later turn out to be unnecessary. The problem is that a doctor won't be able to tell beforehand.

False negatives

Much more worrying is the few 'false negatives' that screening will pick up: this is where the mammogram shows no cancer when there is actually one there. The true number of false negatives is hard to determine, because women who have negative mammograms are not subjected to further tests.

False negatives can happen when mammography is used by itself as a test for breast cancer – when this happens, it can miss 15 per cent of tumours. This can occur if the breast tumour is, for example, a cellular one, where there is not much of a fibrotic skeleton to provide enough contrast on the X-ray. Mammography should ideally be used alongside other techniques such as a clinical examination by a doctor (clinical examination, however is *not* part of the UK Screening Programme), monthly BSE and even ultrasound. Ultrasound can reveal if an abnormal mammogram is actually a *cyst*.

Screening results

It is estimated that out of 200 women eligible for screening, only one will require treatment for cancer: twenty out of the 200 women screened will have an abnormality requiring further assessment; three out of the twenty referred on will need a biopsy; and one out of the three having a biopsy will have cancer. Nineteen of the twenty will *not* have cancer. The main disadvantage to screening, apart from the unnecessary biopsies on some women, is the possible over-treatment of non-invasive cancers that may stabilise or be capable of spontaneous regression. (Some women will have a mastectomy for disease that would have been treatable by lumpectomy, or if the cancer had been left alone, would have caused no harm anyway.) Mammography is extremely useful for very large breasts where BSE may be difficult or impossible, but it may be useless for very small breasts.

Where to find screening

If the National Screening Programme has not yet been set up in your neighbourhood, your GP can refer you to the nearest 'early diagnostic unit', or well woman screening clinic, where, hopefully, they will have the latest up-to-date breast- and pelvic-screening services. Or you can ring your Community Health Council (listed in your local telephone directory), or contact the Women's National Cancer Control Campaign (see the list of addresses on p.278) for details of your nearest screening.

The interval between screenings

What is the right interval between screenings? A Swedish study concluded that annual screening should pick up 90 per cent of cancers; two-yearly screening should pick up 80 per cent; and three-yearly screening, 70 per cent. That means that two to three out of every ten women with breast cancer may be missed when screened every three years. The 'ideal' screening interval is hotly debated by doctors, but it should reflect a compromise between the high cost of running an annual screening programme and the risk of a cancer developing between screening intervals (known as an 'interval cancer').

Can mammography cause cancer?

There has been some argument that mammography itself, being an X-ray technique, could give you breast cancer. In theory it is more of a risk to a woman under the age of thirty-five as her breasts are more vulnerable due to greater hormonal activity. The radiation dose given off by a mammogram is extremely low, and the benefits of screening far outweigh any radiation risk. Screening is justified because 85 per cent of women with disease confined to the breast which is discovered and treated at an early stage survive for at least five years, and many survive much longer, without a recurrence. At present, one of the only ways substantially to reduce the number of deaths from breast cancer is to find it before there are symptoms – that is, at an early stage.

Screening for women after mastectomy

A woman who has had a mastectomy still needs to have her normal breast screened annually. In between screenings she should regularly examine her breast, *and* the mastectomy site, even if a breast reconstruction has been done.

Screening advice

As regards mammography, remember that any 'negative' result applies to *now*, this minute, and not to tomorrow. Not all breast cancers show up on X-ray, and some cancers show no changes in the early stages, which is why monthly BSE is so important.

RECURRENCE

Breast cancer, like endometrial cancer, has a tendency to recur in later years. Whatever form of therapy is used, 5-10 per cent of women will suffer a local recurrence either as a nodule on the mastectomy scar on the chest wall (if a mastectomy has been performed), or as a recurrence in the same breast. This could be either a true recurrence or a new focus of the cancer elsewhere in the same breast. To prevent a recurrence, a woman may be put on hormone therapy. Low doses of radiation may be suggested to stop the ovaries from functioning – but as this is *permanent*, and anti-hormone drugs (such as Zoladex) have only a temporary effect, a woman may be better off with the hormone therapy. The problem with Zoladex is that it is not yet widely available and is expensive.

Women who have a higher risk of recurrence are those who have surgery other than a mastectomy. Michael Baum, Professor of Surgery at King's College Hospital, London, believes that 15 per cent of women who've had cancer in one breast will get cancer in the other breast *if they live long enough* – but the risk works out to be less than 1 per cent a year. Sixty per cent of recurrences happen in the first three years after initial treatment; 20 per cent within the next two years; and 20 per cent in later years.

A woman should be examined frequently in the first five years following treatment and continue to be checked by her GP as often as he/she recommends in subsequent years. It is not easy to avoid becoming obsessed with looking for signs of a recurrence; try, however, to keep a watchful eye on yourself *without* becoming neurotic.

The following symptoms *could* signal a recurrence, or they

could be the result of arthritis, influenza, the menopause or even the common cold:

1. Changes in the affected breast or breast scar, such as inflammation or thickening.
2. Persistant pain in the breast, shoulder, hip, lower back or pelvis.
3. Persistent coughing or hoarseness.
4. Digestive disturbances lasting for several days, including nausea, vomiting, diarrhoea, heartburn.
5. Loss of appetite or unexplained weight changes.
6. Changes in menstrual cycle or flow.
7. Persistent dizziness, blurred vision, severe or frequent headaches, difficulty in walking.

Ask your doctor what else you should be looking for, and how often you should be examined.

SURVIVAL

Doctors consider the condition of the armpit nodes to be the most important factor for predicting long-term survival after breast cancer: survival is best when no nodes are involved, and worst when four or more nodes are involved. Eighty per cent of women with small tumours and no nodes involved get past five years.

Survival also depends on the intrinsic malignancy of the tumour, and the stage at which it was diagnosed, which makes a stronger case for earlier diagnosis. Breast cancers can vary tremendously in the way that they grow: some grow and spread very early, while others take several years to grow and spread. A carcinoma in situ (see p.71) may never progress at all, or it may stabilise, or even regress. In fact, women with one of the larger types of tumours – over 6 cm (2.5 inches) in size – may have a better survival rate. Some breast cancer patients live to a ripe old age and die of other causes, because their cancer is so slow-growing, with cells that are only *slightly* different from normal ones.

Breast cancer has the third best prognosis for survival after cervical and endometrial cancers. The latest national figures for England and Wales show a five-year survival rate of 64 per cent. Advances in treatment have achieved only modest increases in survival time, one of them being a 30 – 40 per cent reduction in the risk of dying over five years for pre-menopausal women with positive lymph nodes – and it might be for a long as ten years. Says Professor Baum: 'If we did nothing, one woman in ten would be alive in ten years; if we did something, five women out of ten would be alive in ten years. Only 35 per cent of breast cancer is cured by orthodox therapy, but the quality of life of survival time has been greatly improved'.

Remember that survival or 'prognosis' times are statistical terms of probability. Doctors do not like to give them, because they cannot possibly predict how an individual will react to cancer. When pushed to do so by family and friends, doctors will fall back on 'median' life expectancy figures (see p.34), but these are only a rough, general guideline.

THE ORTHODOX FUTURE

Because the cause(s) of breast cancer is/are not understood, there is no immediate prospect for prevention; and although a lot of money is being spent on early detection, more money needs to be directed at the possible reasons *why* it occurs. But where to *start* is the problem.

One study currently taking place at Guy's Hospital, London, is trying to discover if benign breast disease is related to malignant disease. Dr Jack Cuzick, an ICRF statistician, is following up 40,000 women with benign breast disease.

In the future there may be a drug to mimic the favourable effects that early pregnancy has on the risks of breast cancer. This would be a contraceptive pill with protective progestogen in it, but before that occurs, trials will need to be done to ensure that it *is* a protective agent; and then further trials would be necessary to compare one control group to another. All of this may take another twelve years.

It may be possible to change a particular hormone pattern in a women who appears to be at a higher risk – trials now going on with the drug Depo Provera may achieve this. And tamoxifen may prove useful as a preventative after all. At some point in the future, where there is a strong family risk, it may be possible to change a deficient gene inherited by a baby when it is still in the womb (technically known as 'reversing oncogene activation').

WHAT YOU CAN DO TO HELP YOURSELF

- Practise breast self-examination (BSE) every month (see p.121).
- Keep your weight down: the incidence of breast cancer that develops post-menopausally increases in overweight women.
- If you can, have your babies young, before the age of thirty, and complete your family before you turn thirty-five: one specialist believes that early pregnancy changes the balance of hormones in a 'once and for all' way, by allowing the breast to shed many of its epithelial cells.
- Cut down on all fats in your diet.
- Avoid or cut down on caffeine and alcohol, as both have been linked with breast cancer. Alcohol combined with heavy smoking is particularly risky.
- If you use the contraceptive pill, make sure that you take a low-dose, 'combined' brand.
- Have your partner keep an eye out for breast lumps: believe it or not, it is often boyfriends or husbands who discover lumps first.

THE COMPLEMENTARY APPROACH

Neither orthodox nor complementary therapies have cracked breast cancer; overall, the survival rate has remained the same for years. So few women have tried complementary in preference to orthodox therapies that nothing yet can be said about their relative success or failure. But it is worth noting that a breast cancer that is not treated at all could become an open, ulcerating wound. If you are diagnosed as having a breast cancer in its early stages, you could opt to have just the lump or tumorous portion of the breast removed (if possible), to be followed by more orthodox treatment, or alternative treatment, or ideally a combination of both.

Diet

Follow the anti-cancer diet; or you might want to try one of the other dietary approaches suggested on pp.183 – 193. Avoid meat and poultry that has been treated with hormones, as breast cancer is hormone-receptive. Buy organically reared meat whenever possible.

Vitamins

Take all the vitamins and enzymes mentioned on pp.197 – 203; in particular, vitamins C and A. Go easy on vitamin E as in large doses it can possibly stimulate hormone activity.

Minerals

Take all the minerals mentioned on pp.203 – 205; and in particular, take a minimum of 100 mg of selenium a day, as research shows that it may inhibit the breakdown of fats into cancerous by-products. Selenium is a trace element found in the soil and in water.

Supplements

Take GLA, bromelain, probiotics, Iscador (see p.208). Avoid ginseng as it is a hormone stimulant.

Herbal remedies

These are made up for the individual, but you might be given remedies including Poke Root, Wild Yam (both clean out the lymphatic system), Wild Violet leaves (believed to be a cancer inhibitor) and Red Clover, but not if there is active ulceration. Mistletoe may also be given in the form of a tea, but it should be steeped overnight in cold water (see p.229). Packs of herbs containing Red Clover and Wild Violet leaves may be used as a poultice.

Homoeopathy

There are many different homoeopathic remedies for breast cancer based on an individual patient's emotional state and symptom pattern (see pp.230 – 236). Hemlock, for example, is given for lumpy breasts associated with grief; while phosphoric acid may be prescribed to increase energy levels after chemotherapy treatment.

Other things you may want to try

Detoxification (p.218); acupuncture, particularly with Chinese herbs (p.236); counselling, relaxation, bio-feedback, breathing exercises (p.244); meditation, visualisation and spiritual healing (p.250).

Part Three

Alternative/ Complementary Treatments

9

The Alternative Approach to the Four Women's Cancers

Alternative therapies for cancer are any treatments besides the orthodox ones of surgery, chemotherapy, radiotherapy and hormone therapy. For the purposes of this book, they include mainly diet, vitamin and mineral supplementation and other supplements, Iscador, detoxification, herbalism, homoeopathy, acupuncture, relaxation, meditation, visualisation and spiritual healing. Counselling is found on both sides of the fence. Some alternative therapists believe that it is orthodox medicine which is the 'alternative' approach, as therapies like acupuncture, herbalism and spiritual healing have been around for thousands of years.

When alternative therapies are used alongside orthodox treatments, with the common aim of helping the individual's return to health, they are called 'complementary' therapies. It should be clearly understood that complementary therapies do not interfere with orthodox treatments when they are taken together, but rather enhance them. Although it is ultimately up to the individual to choose the treatment(s) that best suit her, I do not believe it is wise to 'use' alternative treatments as a replacement for orthodox treatments; rather, alternative treatments will be discussed as a 'complementary' option, not as an 'either/or' option, which the word 'alternative' conveys to many people.

You may have heard the term 'holistic', meaning to take into account the whole person on all levels, which include the physical, emotional, mental and spiritual levels. Not all complementary therapies are holistic: a specialised dietary approach, for instance, is not holistic, as it takes into account only the physical level. Herbalism, homoeopathy and acupuncture *are* holistic, because they address the individual on most levels.

But why should a woman need other treatment for her cancer apart from the orthodox treatments? Orthodox medicine is very good at treating 'acute' conditions such as medical emergencies, but its track record with 'chronic' conditions like cancer is not as successful: apart from an improvement in results with a couple of rare cancers like Hodgkin's disease, survival statistics for cancer treated by orthodox methods haven't changed much in the last thirty years. There is also a limit to how much surgery, chemotherapy and radiotherapy a body can tolerate: many times orthodox treatments must be stopped at a certain point, while the patient continues to live with her cancer. Orthodox treatments are aggressive, often with toxic side effects, and these can create complications with are sometimes fatal in themselves. The patient is treated on a physical level only, and must submit passively to what is being prescribed.

COMPLEMENTARY THERAPIES

Complementary therapies are gentle and have no side effects. Complementary therapists (and many orthodox doctors) believe that the mind and body interact and affect each other – that mental stress and emotional turmoil can damage physical health by weakening the body's immune system and that physical ailments can have emotional and mental consequences. Complementary therapists do not believe that you can treat physical illness without considering the whole being.

Although mental and emotional stress are not seen as automatic precursors to cancer, negative emotions have been linked to the onset of disease by one school of thought since the second century AD. We have often heard of people who have 'worried' themselves ill, and it is certainly possible to measure the chemical changes that occur in the body (for example, alterations in the levels of stress hormones, adrenalin and steroids) when a person is psychologically agitated.

Many therapists view the brain as the centre for the

production or repression of powerful chemicals which directly affect personal well-being. A study in the *Journal of Psychological Medicine* (1982) on women with breast cancer showed that those with a good psychological response to their condition had higher levels of gamma globulin (the serum which builds up disease-fighting antibodies) in their blood! But a deeper understanding of how the neuro-endocrine system interacts with the immune system is needed before stronger claims can be made. Complementary therapies are gentle and have no side effects.

Complementary therapists view cancer not as a localised disease, but as the final symptom in a lengthy degenerative process. A tumour is merely a symptom of the disease, but not the disease itself. To complementary therapists, cancer does not come out of nowhere but is the result of a slow weakening of the body's immune system over the years, through deficiencies in diet and/or lifestyle. Dr Josef Issels, famous medical doctor and alternative cancer therapist, says, 'A healthy body cannot develop cancer. Before a tumour can grow, the body must be sick. When cancer develops, the body's defences are too weak to resist.'

The orthodox doctors disagree, saying that healthy people *do* get cancer. In order to prove this theory one way or the other, doctors or therapists would first need to do research to determine exactly what the body's natural defence system is, what causes it to break down and how to repair it. No one yet has these answers.

Complementary therapists believe that the body has the ability to heal itself, given the right support. Some believe that the real cause of cancer is not physical but emotional. As one therapist puts it, the environment can weaken an immune system and activate a tendency towards cancer, but it doesn't *cause* cancer; emotionally destructive patterns cause cancer. Orthodox doctors would argue that the link between the mind and the immune system is weak, although many complementary therapists believe that the number of white blood cells and their activities can be influenced by the mind. This is a belief held by, among others, Lawrence Le Shan, who is considered by many to be one of the world's leading authorities on the psychology of cancer. He believes that positive and negative thoughts each lead to the production of very different chemicals by the brain, and that emotions like depression, fear, panic and frustration can lead to the healing resources of the brain not being fully engaged.

Complementary therapies give back to the patient that feeling of being in control, by making her an active participant in her fight for survival. Each alternative therapy tries to accomplish one or more of the following four benefits for cancer patients:

1. To support the body's defences and stimulate the immune system.
2. To cleanse toxic substances from the person's body.
3. To attack the tumour directly.
4. To relieve pain and emotional/mental distress.

Many of the complementary therapies, particularly the holistic treatments, can also help to minimise the side effects of radiation and chemotherapy. One study has shown that terminal breast cancer patients given a combination of chemotherapy and psychotherapy survived much longer than other groups of patients who were given chemotherapy alone, psychotherapy alone, or no treatment at all.

By law, complementary therapists are not allowed to say that they treat cancer: they get around this by treating the *whole* person. Many will refuse to take on a cancer patient unless she consults an orthodox medical doctor as well, as it is he/she who has ultimate responsibility for the patient. The initial diagnosis and the intermittent testing to reveal the state of the disease must rest with the orthodox doctors and their precise, high-technology equipment, as diagnosis by a complementary therapist is not as reliable as an orthodox diagnosis. Likewise, if an 'acute' condition arose, requiring life-saving treatment or immediate symptom relief, the orthodox doctors would be in charge.

Cancer is considered a 'chronic' condition, because it can take many years to develop – similarly, there is no fast or easy cure, and this is never promised by either side. Some complementary therapists hold the view that when the body returns to an improved state of health, the malignancy will often slow down or regress, as they believe that cancer cannot exist in a balanced metabolic state.

There is no simple answer as to whether complementary therapies will definitely help with cancer – a change in diet or lifestyle by itself may not automatically lead to recovery or remission, but at the very least the patient will experience improved well-being, a calmer state of mind and a reduction in any pain or symptoms. Complementary therapies may work for some people and not for others; in the same way, orthodox treatments work for some and not for others. It could be said that the failure of some complementary therapies in some cases could have less to do with the therapy itself than with the ability of the practitioner or the condition of the patient when she began treatment: many patients undertake complementary therapies at a late stage in their cancer, or after being debilitated by too much chemotherapy or radiotherapy.

Some patients who have taken nothing but complementary treatment are alive and well long past the survival times predicted by orthodox doctors – but the latter argue that they would have survived anyway, as every cancer has a small percentage of long-term survivors. However, such things are difficult to label: is it a 'cure', a 'remission' or a 'stabilising' when the cancer lives quietly in the body but no longer interferes with it? Many people, whatever course of treatment they try, survive their cancer only to die of something else in their old age.

PROOF FOR COMPLEMENTARY THERAPIES

Some orthodox doctors claim that the way alternative therapies work is by the 'placebo effect', meaning that the therapy works because both the therapist and the patient *believe* that it will. But even the orthodox doctors admit that the placebo effect is a real phenomenon, and that it can be quite strong. Can this really be all there is to complementary therapies?

It is said by the orthodox camp that complementary therapists have no scientific proof that their therapies work as they don't subject their treatments to rigorous controlled trials in the way that orthodox doctors do. According to Professor Baum, all scientists must expose their favoured hypothesis to scientific trials, and that if complementary therapists say that they cannot do so, their treatment claims must stay within the realm of faith rather than that of science. Professor Baum, in fact, does not believe in drawing a line between orthodox and complementary methods. He says, 'A treatment either works, or it doesn't work. I don't care where the remedy comes from, but the laws of evidence must be applied. If you cannot collect evidence scientifically, then you have only a belief system.'

What orthodox doctors would like complementary therapists to do is 'double-blind' trials – this is where one group of patients is given a specific treatment as compared to another group which is not, with neither the doctors giving the treatments nor the patients receiving them knowing who is getting what. Only the person running the trial from behind the scenes knows the score – that way, nobody's 'belief system' can influence the way the trial will go.

However, complementary therapists argue that it is difficult if not impossible for them to do such trials, for the following reasons:

1. It is 'unethical' to have a placebo group, where some patients do not receive the beneficial treatment. All patients coming to a therapist must be treated with the best treatments that the therapist has at his/her disposal.

    One complementary therapist (who is also a medical doctor) argues, 'Has there ever been a "mastectomy" group compared to a "no surgery" group? Certainly not – they wouldn't dare leave a group of breast cancer patients untreated by surgery, and yet orthodox doctors tell us to suspend treatment in one patient group.'

2. It would be difficult to find sufficient numbers of patients to do such tests on, in order to achieve a plausible result. Complementary therapists do not have access to the numbers of patients that orthodox doctors do, as they can treat only the people who come to see them.

3. The complementary approach consists of many aspects – diet, vitamins, supplements, visualisation and so on – and it is impossible to separate them out as they all work together in a 'synergistic' way (this is, the parts of the treatment taken *together* have a stronger effect than if they were each used separately).

4. Complementary therapies are often taken alongside orthodox treatments by patients, so again it is difficult to single out precisely what is working. It could be that the

    alternative remedies and the orthodox treatments are working synergistically with each other.

5. Holistic therapies such as herbalism, homoeopathy and acupuncture are prescribed for an individual by matching specific symptoms and personality to a remedy, thus making it impossible to compare one individual to another, let alone one group to another.

Complementary therapists would argue that they have plenty of case histories by which to measure the success of their treatments, and point to the number of their surviving patients as proof that their therapies work. They would argue that subjective data – how the patient *feels* – may not be important to the scientists, but that it is everything to the patient!

Despite all this, trials are being set up to see if complementary therapies can be tested and measured in some kind of controlled way. The Research Council for Complementary Medicine is subsidising a number of research projects designed to test the effectiveness of various therapies. In June 1986 the Institute of Cancer Research and the Bristol Cancer Help Centre began comparing the five-year survival rate and the rate of recurrence in those breast cancer patients who are following the Bristol method with those who are receiving orthodox treatment. Results will be published in 1991.

In November 1988 an evaluation of holistic cancer treatments which are in use throughout Europe was started under the auspices of the Association of New Approaches to Cancer (ANAC) and involves seventy therapists. When the results of these and other complementary therapy trials are in, it may be that the orthodox doctors will have the 'scientific proof' that they demand. Although there is not yet a great deal of hardcore evidence, it doesn't mean that there never will be. And perhaps it would be fairer to devise a way to test complementary therapists that is more in harmony with their treatment of patients, instead of forcing them to fit into the orthodox testing mould.

Despite all the arguments as to what is working and what isn't, there is no question that at the very least, complementary therapies add greatly to the quality of life, simply because they address much more than just the tumour itself. If there are deficiencies in a person's diet or lifestyle, these will be pointed out and the individual will be helped to correct them. If a patient is overcome by feelings of fear, despair and helplessness, there are many things that the therapists can do to help the patient alleviate such feelings. The approach is a positive, gentle one that lifts a person out of her 'patient' role and gives her some weapons with which to fight the cancer.

USING ORTHODOX AND ALTERNATIVE THERAPIES TOGETHER: THE COMPLEMENTARY APPROACH

Patients who wish to use any of the alternative/complementary therapies mentioned in the following chapters alongside their orthodox treatments should first establish a proper diagnosis at the outset with an orthodox doctor. It is also a good idea to have as much of the tumour removed as possible: this is called 'de-bulking', and even alternative therapists make a case for it, especially for an 'in situ' cancer, which is localised (in one place).

It is also very important to establish with a sympathetic orthodox doctor just how much time you have before the cancer grows or spreads: this may not matter so much if you are combining treatments, but if you want to try alternative therapies *before* orthodox treatments, you will need to be very aware of how your particular cancer can be expected to act. For example, a woman with CIN (see p.81) or a small, non-invasive breast lump would have more time to think about and try different treatments than a woman with stage 2 ovarian cancer (see p.53) or an endometrial cancer.

Whether your choice of treatment is orthodox or complementary or both, it is important to remember that healing is something a person does for herself: treatment can only stimulate the body to get it to the point where it can heal itself. A complementary therapist concentrates on removing blockages to the healing process. But complementary therapies work slowly, over a long period of time, and are not good at tackling aggressive, fast-growing tumours – for these, orthodox treatments should be the main approach. Complementary therapies will help by reducing the side effects of the orthodox treatments, and by strengthening the immune system. Or, if you feel that you are on a downhill slide, use orthodox treatments first, before slowly building your immune system up with complementary therapies.

As to how to choose which therapies to try, that must be left for each woman to decide, but the following chapters in this book will help you. Some people will swear that a particular therapy 'saved' them, but no one can plan a course of treatment for you. Everyone is different, and what works for one woman will not work for another. The solution seems to be to make full use of all the available options in a way that suits your personality and needs.

HOW TO CHOOSE A COMPLEMENTARY THERAPIST

First of all you should be just as critical of a complementary therapist as you would be of an orthodox doctor – there are good and bad ones in each field. You could start by asking your GP to recommend one, as many GPs are interested in complementary therapies. The ideal is to find an orthodox doctor who uses complementary therapies, or a complementary therapist who started with an orthodox medical background.

To find out more about a particular therapy before pursuing it, you could always ring your local branch of the British Holistic Medical Association. Then contact the professional body of the therapy that you are interested in (see the list of addresses on p.276)

The number of complementary therapists is estimated to be increasing by 15 per cent every year, but as many as half of all such practitioners are not registered with a professional association at all. Protect yourself from the few unscrupulous therapists, or even the well-meaning amateur, by sticking to those therapists registered with an accredited body. The Bristol Cancer Help Centre and the Association for New Approaches to Cancer (ANAC) have links with both orthodox and complementary practitioners and may be able to recommend one in your area.

Many of the alternative health bodies themselves belong to either the Council for Complementary and Alternative

Medicine (CCAM) or the Institute of Complementary
Medicine (ICM) – see the list of addresses on p.276. The
CCAM tends to stick with strictly scientific explanations of
complementary therapies, whereas the ICM takes the spiritual
aspects of complementary therapies more into account.

Dealing with your chosen therapist

Ask your chosen therapist if he has treated your particular
problem before and, if so, ask to speak to some of his other
patients. Avoid any therapist who blames you for your illness,
or who insists that his/hers is the only route to follow – a
combination of therapies is always wisest and safest. Make sure
that you understand your treatment and why your therapist is
recommending it. Ask your therapist to stay in touch with your
GP. Allow more time for complementary therapies to take effect
than for orthodox therapies.

Some complementary therapists, and some complementary
therapy centres, hammer home the idea that ill health is the
result of a person's irresponsible attitude or incorrect lifestyle.
This can lead to a woman blaming herself for her cancer, which
is something to be avoided – a cancer patient has quite enough
to worry about without piling on the guilt. If you feel that this
is happening to you, change your therapist or treatment centre.
If you come to feel that your cancer does seem connected to a
deep emotional problem, make sure that you use this
information in a *positive* way, not a negative one.

The cost of complementary therapies is not cheap, and if
money is a problem, find a therapist with a sliding scale of fees.
Some professional bodies like The British Herbal Medicine
Association have a training school where you can be treated
cheaply by a student under professional supervision.

BRIDGING THE GAP

Some hospitals, like St Mary's in London, are bridging the gap
between orthodox and complementary treatments: the hospital
team has close links with the British Holistic Medical Association, and it preaches an enlightened awareness of both

orthodox and complementary methods, stressing the need for high-quality therapists on both sides. Although Professor Baum may be one of complementary medicine's most outspoken critics, he also sees a need for meeting 'in the middle'.

Throughout the world, there are alternative therapists who have had orthodox medical training, who possibly embody the best that both sides can offer. A list of the first orthodox doctors to use alternative therapies would have to include such people as Dr Hans Nieper (nutritional therapy), Dr Hans Moolenburgh (non-toxic cancer therapies), Professsor Werner Zabel and Dr Werner Kollath (nutritional medicine), Dr Milan Brych (immunotherapy of cancer), and perhaps the best-known and most influential – Dr Josef Issels. Some of these men are no longer alive, but their theories and treatments live on.

In the USA many complementary therapists have a scientific or medical background and are doing exciting cancer research that appears to hold great promise. This includes:

- An attempt to help the immune system fight cancer through the development of a 'de-blocking' agent, which counteracts a substance thought to be produced by some cancers to 'block' the immune system. The work is being done by Dr Laurence Burton at his clinic in the Grand Bahamas.
- An attempt to convert cancer cells back into normal ones by supplying a missing protein peptide called antineoplaston, which is the work of Dr Stanislaw Burzynski.
- The development of a drug called hydrazine sulfate which, while not a cancer cure, seems to be able to block a cancer tumour's ability to debilitate the body. This is the work of Dr Joseph Gold.
- The discovery of a microbe called progenitor cryptocides, (PC) found naturally in the body by Drs Issels and Gerlach, which is being further studied by Dr Virginia Livingston Wheeler. PC appears to change its form under the influence of a carcinogen and turns normal cells into cancer cells. Dr Wheeler is working on a PC vaccine to immunise cancer patients against PC infection: if her theories are correct, this could be the forerunner of a universal cancer vaccine.

10

The Bristol Cancer Help Centre

The Bristol Cancer Help Centre was founded in 1980 as a pilot project for a new approach to the treatment of cancer. It deserves a chapter all to itself because it was the first self-help cancer centre in the UK and it has served as a model for most of the other cancer centres and self-help groups. In 1983 it opened its new premises in Grove House in Bristol, and it has recently been renamed simply 'The Cancer Help Centre'.

Each of the three co-founders brought a different but complementary ability to the centre: Dr Alec Forbes brought a knowledge of the physical functions of the body; Penny Brohn a knowledge of the behavioural sciences, alternative medicine and oriental philosophy; and Pat Pilkington an understanding of the way that body and spirit can interact in spiritual healing. Dr Forbes had been an NHS doctor until he became disillusioned with what he saw as orthodox medicine's failure to deal adequately with chronic diseases like cancer. He began to realise that psychological and nutritional factors had a role to play in initiating disease.

The centre was founded on the following principles:

1. That the centre should be holistic in its treatments.
2. That the patient has a right to assume some responsibility for his/her own health.
3. That a lifestyle designed to prevent cancer from occurring or recurring may be made available.
4. That patients may be informed about the safe and gentle therapies that could be used to counteract disease and enhance health, and be provided with a safe, loving and

supportive environment in which they can tune in to and identify their own needs, and begin the process of self-exploration through which they can understand the role of illness in their life and what they need to regain health, balance and control.

5. That the centre should be a non-profit making organis-ation, with the work of the centre being easily available to everyone.

The centre concentrates on those gentle approaches to cancer that its founders believe were swept away by the high technology revolution in twentieth-century medicine. Their programme involves a week's training in which the patient consults with doctors, counsellors, nutritionists and healers. The centre is educational rather than medical and is not equipped to cope with very sick patients.

THE CENTRE'S METHOD

Each patient meets up with a doctor for medical counselling; her medical history is reviewed and any queries answered in an unhurried atmosphere. This may result in the patient wishing to make changes in her lifestyle and/or diet. The doctors and trained nurses at the centre often give a woman the courage to ask her specialist questions that she has held back, or help a person to come to a decision about some major treatment.

Each visitor with cancer can also talk through her own problems, life-enhancing possibilities and unexpressed creativity with a counsellor, either individually or in a group with other cancer patients, and joins in groups to learn about self-exploration, self-knowledge and methods of self-healing. Patients not only learn new ways of living, but also put some thought into how they would like to die. There are two separate options: a one-day 'introductory' programme, and a five-day residential stay. The one-day visit provides all the necessary information, whereas the five-day stay provides a much deeper experience of the information provided.

The centre recommends a mostly raw, mostly vegan diet (see the anti-cancer diet, p.186), teaches concepts of good nutrition and believes in vitamin and mineral supplementation. Diet and supplementation are not seen by the centre as tackling cancerous growths directly, but as supportive treatment do help the body heal itself. The centre also teaches various ways to relax the body and the mind – relaxation techniques, biofeedback, deep breathing and meditation – and a way to focus the mind positively on fighting the cancer, known as 'visualisation'. Spiritual healing is also available, and a belief in God is not a necessary prerequisite for taking part. Art therapy is used to unlock a patient's stifled creativity and release potential – it is also employed as a counselling tool, for the products of the right hemisphere of the brain (which represents creativity) are deemed to give quicker insight into any underlying causes of cancer than the 'defending' left hemisphere (which represents rational thought).

It is suggested that suppressed energy can *itself* cause a cancer in some cases. The centre believes that a lack of creative outlets for some people may contribute to their cancer – if, for instance, they have gone through their life with their creative 'life force' suppressed or stifled by ambitious parents, rigid educational establishments or their career choice. In the same way, it is believed that creativity may be part of the *healing* process. But cancer as 'foiled creative fire' (Lawrence Le Shan's words) is only one model, out of the hundreds which the centre uses, which may have resonance with a particular patient.

Patients at the centre make up their own package of treatments from what is offered, according to their needs and interests. There is no one Bristol programme, because the centre doesn't believe that the same advice can apply to everybody. The 'toolbox' metaphor is relevant here: some tools in the box will be used, while others will remain in the box.

The centre's approach in no way conflicts with orthodox cancer treatments; its treatments may be used in a complementary way alongside orthodox ones and can be continued after orthodox treatments have stopped. The centre's methods can even be used when no orthodox treatment has been offered in the first place. It believes in the synergistic effect created by using more than one kind of therapy at the same time. Many of its patients have had or are receiving hospital treatment, but seem to tolerate orthodox treatments better and suffer fewer physical and emotional side effects after a visit to the centre.

However, the staff at the centre don't believe that orthodox medicine goes far enough in mobilising the inner resources of the patients themselves – and that aggressive external attacks on cancer are often more traumatic than the disease itself. They don't encourage patients to take the Bristol route only, but if a patient insists in doing so, they respect her wishes. Some patients who have used only Bristol's methods have survived; others have not. The centre holds the view that conventional treatments should be used if a patient's life is in immediate danger, if the patient so wishes. Again, it is a matter of the patient's choice – the centre has no 'policy' statement to offer!

What the Bristol staff do believe is that no one person or institution has all the answers, and with that in mind they have gathered together information about many different cancer treatments which is available on request. They reiterate that the treatments they propose are safe and have no side effects.

The patient's family

The centre is not only for cancer patients, but for their family and friends as well. The staff recognise that the loved ones of a cancer patient are just as stressed and confused as the patient, and so they encourage you to bring along a friend or a close family member to share in the learning experience.

Case Study – BRISTOL CANCER HELP CENTRE
In February 1985, at the age of fifty-three, June Rogers visited her doctor because she was losing weight, felt excessively tired and was passing blood in her urine. Tests such as an intravenous pyelogram showed nothing, but a cystoscopy (direct visualisation of the bladder) revealed an egg-sized tumour in her bladder. A biopsy of the tumour confirmed squamous cell carcinoma. During a second cystoscopy as much cancerous material as possible was removed.

Ten years earlier June had undergone a total hysterectomy, at which point a cyst was discovered on her right ovary. It was diagnosed as an adenocarcinoma and removed. This was followed by radiotherapy treatment. The doctors couldn't decide if the new bladder tumour was a secondary from her ovarion tumour or a new primary. June herself is convinced that it was a new primary, caused by the original radiotherapy treatment.

The specialist told her that she would need her bladder removed. June refused; she knew that she could deal with the tumour herself, mainly through spiritual healing. She put down her excellent recovery

*from ovarian cancer to all the healing she had received during the
early part of her illness. Giving herself three months to clear the
bladder tumour, she visited the Bristol Centre which she'd heard
about through a nursing friend and a television programme.*

*At the centre she learnt about diet and vitamin/mineral sup-
plementation, which made her feel much stronger physically. She
stuck to the Bristol Diet for four months and now modifies it to suit
herself. After a year she cut back on her vitamins, and she now senses
when she needs a particular one. Counselling was new to June too,
and it helped her to know herself better, resulting in a little less loving
of everyone else and a little more loving of herself. This meant it was
now easier for her to draw boundaries, so that she wasn't so constantly available to others. She learnt to 'image' as well, imagining
a fish swimming around in her bladder, taking big chunks of her
tumour away.*

*But June's main weapon was spiritual healing (see page 254).
As it turned out, she did heal herself in three months: when she
returned for her third cystoscopy it was discovered that there was very
little tumour left. All cystoscopies since that time have shown the
bladder to be completely healed, with only a small scar to show where
the tumour once was. Her specialist wonders if it was his attempt to
remove as much cancerous material as possible during the second
cystoscopy that saved her — however, he is also the first to admit that
any partial resection performed via a cystoscope would not constitute
a complete medical treatment of this condition. Her own GP feels
very strongly that June's own self-healing efforts changed the course
of her disease.*

Case Study – BRISTOL CANCER HELP CENTRE
*In December 1975 Diana Thompson discovered that she had breast
cancer. She was forty. She was immediately given a mastectomy, and
all was well until 1981, when her health began to deteriorate and she
was taken back into hospital. A thorocotomy was performed (an
operation involving the opening of the chest) which revealed multiple
secondaries in the lungs, lymph nodes and tissue around the heart.
She was very ill after this operation, and emotionally shattered by the
diagnosis.*

*At this point she and her husband heard about the Bristol Cancer
Help Centre. A few months later, when she was well enough to
attend, she launched herself into the recommended therapies. She
discovered a tremendous feeling of peace and hope at the centre, and*

felt that she was no longer struggling alone. Although she knew that not everyone attending the course recovered physically, she discovered that everyone who did attend felt considerably helped by all the time, concern and love given to them by various staff members.

Diana was encouraged by the centre to carry on taking the tamoxifen recommended by her specialist. She was slowly gaining strength from her new way of life until she had a temporary setback in October 1985: another secondary tumour was found and removed from her stomach muscle. In July 1986 it was discovered that the cancer had spread to her liver. At this point she was taken off the tamoxifen as it didn't appear to be containing the cancer.

Diana had heard about Iscador and wanted to try it. Her doctor supported her in this, because he felt that Western medicine could do nothing else for her. He didn't tell Diana, but he felt that she had only two months to live. Diana has been on Iscador since mid-1986, and is feeling fit and well on it. Both her doctor and her specialist are amazed – it is now over eight years since lung secondaries were diagnosed, and over three years since liver secondaries were found. The only other therapy that Diana sets great store by is spiritual healing, which she receives weekly. She also takes part in a meditation group and visits her local cancer support group.

SUCCESS RATE

You may wonder, 'If I go to the Cancer Help Centre, what are my chances?'. The answer would be, 'We don't know – nobody knows.' There have been well-documented cases of remission, and the centre's staff believe that any one of their visiting patients could be the next remission. There have also been some complete cures, but mostly there is improved quality of life through positive changes in diet and lifestyle. The message seems to be that patients may well affect their own body through an enhanced mental/emotional state, and they are encouraged to fight for remission.

Many patients claim to have arrested or controlled their cancer through the Bristol approach, but this is difficult to prove in a statistical way as the centre hasn't been around long enough to produce hard statistics. In a few years there may be facts and figures when the results of two separate research projects in conjunction with the Imperial Cancer Research Fund become known. What the centre can produce right now, though, is some dramatic case histories.

The centre encourages each patient to take positive action and not to be a 'helpless victim' – in fact, to shrug off the role of passive patient and to take on that of active healer for oneself. The staff firmly believe that the 'compliant' patient has the worst prognosis of all, and that 'difficult' patients do best – that is, those who fight and do not give in, even if it means disagreeing with doctors and therapists.

Diet and vitamins apart, the centre's treatments are more directly aimed at healing the patient on the emotional, mental and spiritual levels. Apart from Iscador treatment (see p.213), which is now on offer at Bristol, no complementary physical treatments are used there to fight a tumour directly. As the centre's therapies are often taken alongside orthodox medical treatments, it is these which are fighting the tumour on a direct physical level.

11
Diet, Vitamins and Supplements

A diet high in the nutrients required by the body is the main weapon used by complementary therapists to fight cancer *physically*. Often extra amounts of certain vitamins and minerals are recommended, as well as certain supplements, like enzymes, GLA and bromelain, which will be mentioned later. Herbalism, homoeopathy and acupuncture also have physical effects, but they are must more subtle. Immuno-stimulants like Iscador produce a physical effect, but they are substances which must be administered by a doctor or qualified therapist. Diet is certainly one area where a woman can do much to help herself.

DIET

A sound diet isn't a guarantee of perfect health, but there is proof that unbalanced eating can upset the body and create conditions in which disease and tumours can thrive. In fact, Sir Richard Doll, the Oxford-based cancer researcher, claims that faulty nutrition is responsible for an estimated 35 per cent of cancer mortality. For some patients a faulty diet may have been involved in helping to start a cancer, while for many more cancer patients this will not be true.

So does a healthy diet keep the immune system strong? We don't know that for sure. Doctors would argue that in countries where there is a lot of malnutrition, there isn't a lot of cancer. There is no evidence, either, that a good diet can make you better once you've *got* cancer, but there is some evidence that it is a preventative.

Complementary therapists believe that if some things in the diet can be shown to be a preventative for cancer, increasing your intake of these things, within reason, is even more beneficial. This is difficult to prove. The converse has more truth in it: that things in the diet which are thought to be carcinogenic, like animal fats, should be reduced even more.

Still, there is certainly every reason to strive for a well-balanced diet, either as a part of a preventative programme to avoid cancer or to help keep the body strong to endure the rigours of orthodox cancer treatments. Chemotherapy treatment can prevent the absorption of nutrients, and well-nourished patients can actually take higher doses of chemotherapy without doing themselves any harm. And – who knows? – perhaps a good diet is doing just that little bit more to combat cancer. Tests on animals have revealed the helpful action of vitamins A and C on cancer tumours, and perhaps soon these tests and others will provide more definite proof of the same action in humans. Complementary therapists would say that we already have this proof – particularly in regard to vitamin C – and that there are many research papers to justify their claims.

On pp. 186 – 193 I give a description of the general anti-cancer diet as advocated by the Bristol Cancer Help Centre and the ANAC. It is followed by a selection of more specific dietary approaches, which you may have heard about and may want to try, but some of them are very difficult to follow without help, and all of them need supervision by a doctor or a therapist. Don't start any kind of special diet without medical approval, as you may not be the best judge of what your constitution can take.

Whatever dietary approach you choose, keep the following points in mind:

• There is no point in trying to stick to a diet that you think is doing you good, if in fact it is making you miserable. Be sensible, and strive for a balance between your physical needs and your emotional needs. Even the Bristol Centre is beginning to believe that your state of mind while you are eating may be the most important factor for extracting goodness from your food. The 'perfect' diet is what feels right and acceptable to *you*, and it shouldn't put any additional stress on the patient or her family.

- Change slowly and don't set too high a standard for yourself to begin with, or you will quickly give up.
- Seek the advice of a nutritionist, naturopath or a doctor or therapist with nutritional training to help you, as everyone has different nutritional needs. What suits you, will not suit another woman – for example, some people need a bit of meat and do not thrive on a vegetarian diet. This has to do with the type of metabolism a person has (see p.196, Dr William Kelley), which may well function better with the kind of proteins, amino acids and so on that only meat can provide. For one thing, meat contains vitamin B12, which is difficult to get in sufficient amounts from other food sources. Some people do very well on a vegetarian diet, while others get more listless, tired and lose weight; these people, in fact, feel more energetic after eating meat. Unfortunately most of today's meat is crammed full of antibiotics and growth promoters – so if you are a cancer patient who, after experimenting, feels she would benefit from some meat, either buy it from an organic butcher or, if this is impossible, eat *small* quantities of the non-organic variety.
- Eat frequent, small meals and chew your food slowly and thoroughly to aid digestion.
- If chemotherapy has given you mouth ulcers, process your food in a blender to make it softer, or use gravies to soften food. Cold foods can be soothing as well.
- If you use cling film, choose one without a 'plasticiser' in its coating, (check the label) as plasticiser's are considered possible carcinogens.
- Don't use aluminium cooking utensils: use glass, enamel, or stainless-steel pots and pans instead. Aluminium can be absorbed into the system, and this is heightened if certain acid fruits like rhubarb are cooked in aluminium pans. There is still controversy surrounding the effects of aluminium, but it is thought to interfere with brain function.
- Throw away left-overs; they will have lost their nutritional value and if you are a cancer patient, you're after the best nutrition that you can get.

THE ANTI-CANCER DIET

The basic anti-cancer diet was devised by Dr Max Gerson, a German emigré to the USA who practised medicine in New York between the 1930s and 1959. He believed that once the body is given the right kind of nutritional help it is capable of cleansing the system of disease.

The rules of the general anti-cancer diet as described mainly by the Bristol Cancer Help Centre and the ANAC are as follows:

Fats

Fats should be kept to a minimum, and this includes all dairy products, margarines and cooking fats and oils; but small amounts of butter, buttermilk, low-fat live yoghurt and the first cold pressing of organic olive oil or grapeseed oil are allowed. It is believed that the liver converts some fats into bile acids, which in turn are converted by bacteria in the gut into tumour growth-promoting material.

The heating of unsaturated fats, including all margarines, may produce carcinogenic substances (though this has not yet been conclusively proved), so if any hot oil is needed, use olive oil (which is monosaturated) – although fried foods really shouldn't be eaten. This is because frying increases the fat content of the food, and excess fats inhibit the production of prostaglandins, which have a protective role. Indeed, cancer scientist Richard Peto has discovered a relationship between breast cancer and fat consumption. The high temperatures used when frying also destroy valuable enzymes.

Remember that the dietary rules that apply to a healthy person apply even more to someone with cancer, as no extra stress should be added to the digestive or immune system. 'Vitaquell' margarine, available from health food stores, is safe for both spreading and cooking.

There is some disagreement about whether live yoghurt is useful, because of the presence of lactic acid, and the fact that many milk products contain growth stimulators – but a small portion a day made from either sheep's or goat's milk is useful for its B-complex vitamins and also for its 'friendly' bacteria, *Lactobacilli*, which promote healthy bacteria in the colon.

Check, however, that the sheep's/goat's milk yoghurt is from untreated animals (that is, reared without growth stimulators).

Vegetables and fruit

Eat vegetables and fruit that are organically grown: that is, grown without pesticides, or artifical fertilisers of any kind. And eat them freshly picked and raw whenever you can.

Green and red peppers, tomatoes, aubergines and potatoes, which are members of the deadly nightshade family, should be avoided, as it is thought they may encourage tumour growth.

There is some evidence that parsnips, celery and parsley should be avoided as well, as they contain psoralen, a possible carcinogen.

Dr Jan De Vries, a cancer specialist, swears by the benefits of beetroot juice, and salads of freshly-grated beetroot, carrot and apple: he claims that these three foods counteract the effects of chemotherapy and radiotherapy, and promote the increase of red and white blood corpuscles, although there is no proof of this. Beetroot, however, *can* help with oxygenation of the blood.

Mushrooms are a fungus and should be avoided, but garlic and onions are recommended because they contain anti-cancer substances. Garlic should be swallowed in small pieces mixed with water before meals, and onions are best eaten raw, if you can stand it! Don't eat garlic or onions with live yoghurt, however, as they can knock out the 'friendly' bacteria in the yoghurt.

Any cooking of vegetables should be done by lightly steaming them. Raw food should be eaten before cooked foods, in order to stimulate the right enzymes in the stomach to help fight the cancer cells.

It may be difficult to buy organically-grown produce, depending on where you live. Sainsbury and Safeway now carry some organic vegetables, and a list of organic suppliers can be obtained from the Soil Association (see the list of addresses on p.191). Or you could advertise for organic vegetables and fruit in your local newspaper – someone may have a surplus of home-grown vegetables and be able to sell or give you some. Don't, however, get neurotic about this; it's far better to eat non-organic vegetables and fruit than none at all. If you can't get organic produce, buy vegetables and fruit as fresh as possible. You could soak them in a mixture of apple cider and water for two hours, to remove any pesticides (unfortunately, vitamins and minerals may also leach out) or you could scrub them.

Grains

There is some evidence that a gluten-free diet should be followed for three months after a diagnosis of cancer, but it may be necessary only for those who prove to have a gluten allergy. Brown rice, millet and buckwheat can be substituted. Wholegrain rice is a good balance between carbohydrates and proteins, helping to balance the body's acid/alkaline level.

Nuts

Nuts should be bought only in season and in their shells. After shelling, the nuts themselves should be washed, and soaked for two hours in a solution of one teaspoon of vitamin C powder to 1 litre (1 ¾ pints) of water. This is to rid them of any possible aflatoxin, a carcinogenic substance resembling a mould that can contaminate nuts that have been badly stored. (This same procedure applies to dried fruits.) A good choice is either cashews or almonds, but avoid peanuts, which aren't nuts at all – they are a kind of bean and are particularly susceptible to aflatoxin.

Beans, peas and seeds

Chick peas, lentils, mung beans and so on are an excellent source of protein, and a rich source of vitamin C and enzymes when sprouted and eaten raw. Try sprouting aduki beans, mung beans, soy beans, lentils, buckwheat and chickpeas, and pumpkin and sunflower seeds. To sprout, put the beans or seeds in a jar, cover them with filtered water, and leave overnight in a warm, dark place like an airing cupboard. Rinse them three times a day in filtered water until they sprout, then put them in the light, and when the sprouts reach 2.5cm (1 inch) in length, they are ready to eat. A more complete description of sprouting is given in Brenda Kidman's book, *A Gentle Way With Cancer* (see the Bibliography on p.296). Sprouts enhance the action of the natural enzymes found in food and in the body. Add sprouts to salads; cooked peas and beans can be added to casseroles and soups.

Avoid brown beans (known as 'ful-mesdames'), alfalfa and sesame seeds because they contain various unhelpful substances.

Eggs

Eggs should be from free-range birds who have not been given antibiotics; the recommended allowance is one to two a week.

Meat

It is normally recommended that meat should be avoided for the first three months of changing your diet: this is because meat is often difficult for cancer patients to digest, it is a source of saturated fat and is likely to contain antibiotics and growth promoters. There could also be chemicals on the grass that the cattle eat. However, if the patient's diet formerly contained a lot of meat, a gradual cut-down may be in order to prevent any reaction to a sudden removal. If you feel out-of-sorts and listless without meat in your diet, you could eat small amounts of organically reared free-range chicken, organic meat or deep-water fish (see p.190).

Some cancer patients fare better on the kind of protein found in meat, especially if they are on chemotherapy or have a low white blood cell count. Meat can help to strengthen the system for chemotherapy, which destroys many red blood cells; so if you feel that you need meat, ask your butcher whether his meat is free from hormone injections (the worst of the additions, especially for female cancer patients). The same applies to chicken. Pork should always be avoided, as it contains a high concentration of toxins and fat. It is interesting to note that free-range animals have been discovered to have 6 per cent fat in their muscle, while factory-bred animals have 26 per cent.

Organically reared meat is from cattle or poultry which are not given growth promotors, steroids (hormones) or antibiotics, and are fed on organically grown, unsprayed feed.

There is some evidence that groups of people such as the Mormons and Seventh Day Adventists, who eat non-animal protein, have less cancer than meat-eating groups of people, although this could be dependent on other factors.

Meat and protein

Some people need the animal protein found in meat in order to stay healthy, as they lack the necessary enzymes to make tissue protein from vegetable protein. To find out if you need meat, ask your doctor for a full blood test that looks at the protein and iron content. In advanced cases of cancer more protein is necessary, as cancer demands protein and will take it from the muscles and organs. PEP (Pure Essential Protein), which is available from health food stores, contains all the necessary amino acids (elements of protein) in powdered form which you can sprinkle on food and into drinks. Eggs, milk and cheese are not good animal protein sources as they are also high in fat. Better alternatives are peas, beans and lentils (see p. 188).

Fish

Fish would give you adequate protein if you didn't want to include meat in your diet. Buy the deep-water varieties, such as cod, mackerel, haddock and salmon, as they are less likely to have absorbed pollutants. Avoid flatfish or shellfish as they live and feed in the more polluted coastal regions and avoid freshwater fish too as they may be affected by river pollution.

Sugar

No sugar is allowed, except occasionally as a 'treat' in the form of a good-quality honey like acacia or heather honey made from an unsprayed crop and bought from a local beekeeper. Sugar can cause you to lose your appetite for nutritious foods, and uses up vitamin B1 when it is metabolised. It also causes the liver and pancreas to struggle to maintain the right insulin/glycogen levels, which in turn uses up vitamins and minerals. Sugar is linked to heart disease too, especially when coupled with a high fat intake.

Salt

Salt should be avoided in all its forms, which include mono-sodium glutamate, used in Chinese cooking; sodium nitrite, used in meat and fish as a curing preservative and sodium phosphate, a wetting agent. Watch out for salt in such foods as Cheddar and Danish Blue cheeses, some stock cubes and bacon. Dried, tinned and packaged foods all have huge amounts of extra salt added.

Sodium and potassium work together in the cells of our body to balance our energy levels, and too much salt kills potassium. In fact, many nutritionists believe that cancer is associated with low levels of potassium, and Gerson, the famous cancer therapist, went so far as to say that the beginning of all chronic disease stemmed from the loss of potassium from the cells. Studies by the World Health Organisation have linked a high-salt diet with cancer. If you feel a craving for salt, try a salt substitute like Ruthmol or Selora, and use herbs like hysssop as flavour enhancers. Spices could irritate the stomach. See p. 203 for foods high in potassium.

Tea/coffee/cocoa/cola

These all contain caffeine and should be avoided. Most types of decaffeinated coffee should be avoided too, because the decaffeinating process uses a chemical which is a potential carcinogen. (Café Hag is one of the few that doesn't.) Coffee, tea, cocoa and cola block the production of prostaglandins. Caffeine interferes with enzyme production, and coffee increases by ten times the formation of nitrosamines in the stomach: these are formed by the stomach acids from nitrites and nitrates, found in our food in the form of preservatives or picked up from agricultural fertilisers. Nitrosamines have been shown to be carcinogenic in tests on animals. Most herbal teas are safe from this point of view, including camomile and lime (linden) blossom, mint, fennel, vervain, elderflower, rosehip, apple and rosehip, rosemary, lemon balm, maté and weak China tea. Avoid sage or ginseng tea, which have an over-stimulating effect on the female hormones. Barley preparations and dandelion coffee are good coffee substitutes and the latter is a good liver stimulator.

Alcohol

One glass of good-quality wine with a meal is permissible, as a little can stimulate prostaglandin formation. Wine from organically grown, non-sprayed vines is available from some major wine shops and health food stores. Avoid cheap wines, as they are often contaminated with chemicals, and all neat spirits should be avoided. Neat alcohol, being fermented sugar, is consumed at the expense of vitamin B6, and is hard on the liver – which is already overworked in a cancer patient as it tries to rid the body of the toxic by-products of cancer cells and of the toxic drugs used in orthodox cancer treatment. Some surveys have shown that people who drink a little live longer than those people who don't drink at all!

Water

Tap water should be avoided because it contains chlorine and fluoride which are enzyme inhibitors, and nitrates which can be converted to nitrosamines (see above). Many people suspect fluoride of being a carcinogen: it is, in fact, a waste product of the aluminium and phosphate fertiliser industries. Its detractors claim that in the regions of the USA and Europe where fluoride has been added to water, cancer rates have risen.

There is disagreement about whether certain store-bought water filters can filter out nitrates, and the consensus is that they cannot. Apart from installing expensive 'reverse osmosis' equipment to filter your tap water (the ANAC should be able to advise you on this), your next best option is to buy the best bottled water, which includes Spa, Volvic, Malvern and Evian. Don't drink too much water with your meals, as it can dilute enzymatic secretions and wash away nutrients before they are absorbed.

Don't forget to drink fresh, unsweetened organic fruit and vegetable juices as well. If you can't buy organic juices, make your own from organic fruit and vegetables.

Processed foods

All processed, packaged and tinned foods should be avoided, not just because of their salt content, but also because of the lack of vitamins and minerals and the presence of preservatives, flavourings, colourings and other additives. We still don't know how many of them could be carcinogenic, how they interact with each other when in the stomach or what their long-term, cumulative effect is. Sodium nitrite, propyl gallate, BHA and BHT are particular ones to avoid. Nitrates and nitrites are used as food preservatives to prevent food poisoning, but it is theoretically possible for these two substances to be converted into nitrosamines in the stomach, which are known to produce cancer in animals. Ask yourself: has the food been ferti-lised/dried/preserved/coloured/flavoured? Frozen foods, while not containing the same amount of additives/preservatives as tinned and packaged goods, are still only a second choice to fresh food which is the cancer patient's ideal.

Here are some of the specific diets that have been devised for cancer patients. Each one of them has its advocates. If you wish to know any more about a particular one, contact the BCHC or the ANAC (see the list of addresses on p.276).

The Bristol Diet

The Bristol Diet was devised by Dr. Alec Forbes and is similar to the anti-cancer diet outlined above, although it is almost entirely vegan and mostly raw, with some yoghurt allowed. It now includes tomatoes and potatoes (which were once forbidden) to make life easier. The Bristol Diet has become more flexible over the years, as the centre now believes that your state of mind with regard to what you're eating may be more important than the things you actually eat. The diet consists basically of 50 per cent vegetables and fruit and 50 per cent wholegrain rice, pulses, nuts, beansprouts and seeds. It allows only enough protein to stimulate the pancreas into producing protein-digesting enzymes (which supposedly go on to destroy the protein coats of the cancer cells, making the cancer cells easier to destroy); but if you crave meat, you can have small portions of organic meat. Protein in general is reduced, but animal protein in particular, as well as fats. Salt, sugar and stimulants are all avoided. It is also important to feel positive about what you are eating.

You are meant to stay on the diet only for a given number of months, and then go on to the maintenance diet which is less rigid. This consists basically of salads, fruit and sprouted seeds, with 50 per cent of intake still raw vegetables, but small amounts of meat are again allowed.

The Hay Diet

The Hay Diet, devised by Dr William Howard Hay in the 1950s, is recommended for cancer patients who have trouble digesting foods like beans (many cancer patients have low stomach acid). It consists of combining foods in certain ways, such as not mixing starches with proteins, as each requires a different acid/alkaline balance for digestion. Starches should be eaten first and then protein, as protein needs to stay in the stomach longer to be digested properly. Fruit is more digestible if eaten an hour after the main meal.

The Allergy-free Diet

The Allergy-free Diet is individually prescribed by a complementary therapist to take into account your allergies, which are determined by a hair and/or a blood analysis. The prototype Allergy-free Diet was devised by Dr Josef Issels in the early 1950s. It usually forbids for a period of time the following foods: dairy products, gluten, alcohol, coffee, tea, chocolate, fried foods, peanuts, pistachios, sesame seeds and sesame oil, and certain vegatables and fruits, depending on the individual.

The Gerson Diet

The Gerson Diet is based on Dr Max Gerson's theory that cancer is a chronic, degenerative disease which disrupts the whole body metabolism, creating a low immune response and generalised tissue damage, especially of the liver. The aim of this diet is to rid the body of poisonous wastes brought on by the breakdown of cancer, and to regenerate the body – particularly the liver – by stimulating self-healing. It is almost entirely vegan, consisting mostly of freshly pressed raw fruit and vegetable juices, plus live yoghurt and juice pressed from the raw liver of freshly killed, organically reared animals. The act of juicing vegetables and fruit releases more enzymes than can be gained from merely eating them raw. There are seven main drinks daily, which are the equivalent of four green salads and three carrot salads. Coffee, tea, alcohol, tap water, smoking and salt are forbidden, but you can drink as much mineral water, herbal tea and fresh fruit juices as you want. Women are not allowed to wear make-up, presumably in order to keep the skin, the largest organ of elimination, clear and free.

Apart from the diet, coffee enemas must be taken regularly to stimulate the liver to eliminate toxins. They are given every four hours at first, day and night. Castor-oil enemas are also used. A description of how to give yourself an enema can be found on p.219. Patients are encouraged to drink large amounts of peppermint tea and take certain supplements, including iodine, potassium, niacin and pancreatic tablets.

Although this approach carries no guarantee of a cure, the Gerson Diet is considered by many complementary therapists to have the best track record of any of the diets for cancer. But it is also one of the toughest anti-cancer regimes, and is only for the most determined – it is hard work and boring, and there is a high drop-out rate. Only one in three patients who try it stick with it long enough for it to do them any good. You will need someone to help you with all the preparations and ideally you should be supervised in a clinical set-up. Even the coffee enemas should be monitored, as you don't want to upset your electrolyte balance or cause heart fibrillation.

A five-year trial on the Gerson Diet of Australian patients in whom cancer had spread to the liver showed several partial remissions. For further information, see under 'Gerson Diet', p.286.

Fasting

Fasting for limited periods of time may be all right for some cancer patients, although it should always be done under supervision. The theory is that the body starts to use up its own tissues during fasting, with the diseased tissue being used up first. Fasting dumps toxins and gives the body a 'spring-clean', while also creating changes in your psychological state: these include a shift in the perception and awareness of things, as well as emotional states becoming more variable, quick-changing and ranging to extremes during the fast.

Fasting in this instance doesn't mean doing without any nourishment at all: vegetable juices, like carrot or a mixture of green vegetables, are taken. The juices are made by processing the vegetables in a juicer, leaving a thick, bulky liquid that is quite filling and not at all like the thin liquids that you buy in cartons or glass jars.

The Grape Diet

The Grape Diet is one of many suggested fruit diets – for grapes, you can substitute oranges, pears, apples or mangoes. The idea is to eat only the fruit when you are hungry, and drink only the freshly pressed juice when you are thirsty. Make sure that the fruit you choose is free from pesticide spray and mould or decay. It is not a good diet for certain cancers like melanoma which thrive on the sugar found in fruit, but breast cancer patients have had a degree of success with it. It should be supervised, and is best done in a clinic over five to seven days. Otherwise, the problem is knowing when to stop.

The Kelley Diet

The Kelley Diet, devised by Dr William Kelley, divides people into around ten different 'types' according to their metabolism, based on the acid/alkaline balance in an individual's body. People are influenced by one of two branches of the autonomic nervous system: either the 'sympathetic' branch, which is acid and stimulating, or the 'parasympathetic' branch, which is alkaline and calming. Everyone is different in the degree to which their bodies are influenced by these branches. Each individual's glands and organs function differently, and differences result in varying chemical and hormonal outputs, which in turn affect personality and physical characteristics. Each metabolic type requires different levels of vitamins, minerals, foods and supplements. Vegetables are alkaline-forming, while meat and grains are acid-forming. It is important for there to be an alkaline residue in the body, and acid-forming foods shouldn't be eaten if the patient has hard tumours.

A therapist must 'type' you, through questionnaire and various tests, before assigning you your 'ideal' diet. This is when you may discover that your system actually needs meat, or understand why you never felt very healthy on certain kinds of diet. The main proponent of this diet in England is Milo Siewert, director of the Bournemouth Centre of Complementary Medicine (BCCM) (see the list of addresses on p.279).

VITAMINS, MINERALS, AND ENZYMES

There are no clear rules about how much extra we might need to take in the way of vitamin and mineral supplements. Do we get all that we need in our food? With the way that food has been sprayed, injected, preserved and processed, it is hard to believe. Cancer patients may have built up chronic deficiencies over the years, as tumours leach vitamins and minerals from the system to promote their own growth. Vitamins and minerals themselves are destroyed by chemotherapy and radiotherapy, and it is known that if extra vitamins are given during treatment the side effects are greatly reduced. There is evidence to suggest that certain vitamins and minerals help the immune system to deal with cancer, and also aid the destruction of cancer-causing substances found in food, but the full role of vitamins and minerals in preventing cancer and helping cancer patients has not been fully established, as most of the studies have been done only on animals.

Vitamins and minerals work together in the body, so if a particular one is missing, it means that others don't get utilised properly. For instance, vitamin D is needed to utilise magnesium and calcium, and in turn magnesium is needed to utilise the B complex vitamins and vitamins C and E. It is important to get nutritional guidance from your therapist, doctor or a nutritionist as to which particular vitamins and minerals you specifically need, which brands, and what the dosage should be.

Taking certain vitamins in isolation can actually leach other vitamins out of the system. Not all brands are of the same quality and, to complicate things further, some vitamins, like C, come in several different forms, and all of the minerals can be bought in different forms. If you are buying vitamins and minerals off the shelf, buy the best that you can afford or the ones that you have been advised to buy, and check the shelf life of each product – large pharmaceutical companies tend to produce their vitamins in big batches only every few years, meaning that many bottles of vitamins may be a few years old. Vitamins can go rancid, and a rancid vitamin can not only leach other vitamins out of your system but have a negative effect as well. Read the labels on each bottle carefully to check on the dosage, and avoid any brands that contain binders, fillers, colouring, yeast, flavours or sugar coatings. These items are difficult to avoid in tablets, so try to stick to powder and capsules.

VITAMINS

Vitamins are important to the body because they make up enzymes, which function as catalysts in nearly all metabolic reactions. Vitamins help in many metabolic processes, such as converting fats and carbohydrates into energy, and help in forming bone and tissue. The theory on vitamins is that more of certain ones can push the body in a healing direction if the body's healing energies are down. Below are some broad guidelines about the vitamins particularly needed to help both prevent and control cancer.

Vitamin A

Vitamin A comes in two forms: the 'active' form derived from animal products such as liver, eggs and fish; and the more 'passive' beta-carotene, which is found predominantly in plants, and which the body converts into vitamin A.

Some of the most persuasive studies regarding the use of vitamins in cancer treatment centre around vitamin A. In animal experiments, vitamin A has prevented the progression of some pre-malignant changes by blocking the action of tumour-causing agents. Apart from stimulating the body's immune system, vitamin A may actually reverse new cancer cells back to normal cells. It seems to prevent cancer cells from making a protein which inhibits the action of the immune system, and also strengthens the mucous membranes against invasion from bacteria and viruses. Vitamin A has also been said to cause regression in epithelial cancers.

The beta-carotene form of vitamin A is found in green, leafy vegetables and yellow-orange vegetables, such as broccoli, cauliflower, sweet potatoes, carrots and Brussels sprouts. Naturally occurring vitamin A is found in fish liver oil. If you are taking vitamin A capsules, make sure that they are in an emulsified form (oil mixed with water) to ensure proper absorption – otherwise, the vitamin will go straight to the liver for storage, instead of circulating in the bloodstream. If the vitamin is not emulsified, take it with a teaspoon of olive oil. Halibut oil capsules are one source of vitamin A; there is also a water-soluble vitamin A in liquid form.

The recommended dosage for cancer patients is 7,500iu, three times a day for a month, and then only one 7,500iu tablet or capsule a day. Up to 50,000iu daily can be taken safely without side effects, but don't exceed that limit as vitamin A can be stored in the body and therefore it's possible to overdose on it. A safer way to take this vitamin is in the form of freshly pressed carrot juice: one glass provides 12,500iu of vitamin A. but don't take both supplements and juice together. One sign that you are taking too much of the beta-carotene form of vitamin A will be if your palms turn yellow – if this happens, cut back on your dosage until the yellowness disappears; this will then be your maintenance dose.

In US trials where a vitamin A-rich diet was given to women a week before they underwent radiotherapy treatment, their response rate to the treatment was improved by 30 per cent. In many countries a low intake of beta-carotene is associated with a higher risk of cancer – women in the ongoing Guernsey study who later developed breast cancer were found to have lower levels of vitamin A. But it could be that low vitamin A is just associated with the *real* cause of cancer.

A derivative of vitamin A is abscissic acid. It is a useful dietary supplement, as it has been shown to slow down the progression of cancerous cells.

Vitamin C

Vitamin C is an anti-oxidant essential for many body functions, helping to metabolise fats, carbohydrates and amino acids, and protecting cell membranes from damage by free radicals. A report in the *British Medical Journal* revealed that lower amounts of vitamin C are found in the white blood cells when the body is stressed. Malignant disorders and bacterial and viral infections all respond to large doses of vitamin C – the vitamin works by strengthening the collagen (the intercellular cement), thus making the body tissues resistant to such things as invasive cancer growths. It also boosts the production of T-lymphocytes, which are blood scavengers. It also detoxifies certain substances in the liver, and helps with healing – especially after surgery.

Vitamin C is the other major vitamin besides vitamin A that blocks the formation of cancer-causing agents, and blocks the conversion of some carcinogens to an active form. Vitamin C is believed to stop the formation of nitrosamines in the stomach (see p.191). Like vitamin A, vitamin C stimulates the immune system. Most cancer patients don't die from cancer, but from infections, haemorrhages and starvation which results from impaired immunity. Vitamin C repairs the immune system. It may also be able to reverse new cancer cells back to normal ones. Studies have shown that it possibly increases the survival time of patients with advanced cancer.

Vitamin C can't *cure* cancer, but it can reduce many of its worst effects as well as minimise the side effects of orthodox treatments. Although the results are good when vitamin C and chemotherapy are taken together, the results are not so good when chemotherapy is taken before vitamin C. Dr Linus Pauling, professor of chemistry and winner of two Nobel prizes, the man who discovered that mega-doses of vitamin C could help ward off the common cold, believes that larger doses of the vitamin help to create antibodies, preserve good health and provide protection against cancer. He claims that cancer patients experience renewed energy and appetite, feel stronger and more alert mentally and can do without painkillers while experiencing no withdrawal symptoms, if they take vitamin C.

Vitamin C cannot be made in the body and cannot be stored there. It is a very unstable vitamin and can be destroyed by exposure to dryness, light, heat, aspirin, smoking and copper utensils. Sun-ripened oranges are a good natural source, as are grapefruit, cauliflower, parsley, cabbage, spinach and Brussels sprouts. Vitamin C foods are best eaten raw; if they are cooked, only a minimum of water should be used, and the water should be boiling before the vegetables are added. But in order to get enough vitamin C you should take a supplement – there is no danger of overdosing, although some people experience diarrhoea at high doses. If this happens, all you need to do is to cut back on the dosage until the diarrhoea stops – this will then be your maintenance dose. Adjusting the dosage also applies if you experience nausea, intestinal gas, heartburn or a mild temperature. At very high doses there may be a danger of depleting the body's supplies of calcium and potassium.

There is some disagreement about what is the correct daily dosage. Dr Pauling believes that a minimum dose for most healthy adults is between 1 and 10g a day, but that between 15 and 20 g taken in three or more divided doses a day is usually safe. He personally believes that taking 10g of vitamin C daily will add another sixteen years to his life – and he is now well into his eighties! If you are under the care of a therapist, ask his/her advice, or start off with 2g daily for two weeks, gradually increasing the dosage to 6g.

Vitamin C should be taken in a form that includes bioflavonoids, which slows down the destruction of this vitamin and aids in its absorption. Ascorbic acid in powder form, is considered a good way to take vitamin C, diluted in orange juice or water. Add some baking powder, says Pauling, to fizz it all up. Other forms of vitamin C include sodium ascorbate, which is more alkaline and useful for highly allergic people, and calcium ascorbate, for those who can't tolerate the other two forms. Avoid capsules or tablets as you could get an allergic reaction while taking large doses of vitamin C in either of these forms: they may contain binders, coating dyes, lubricants and gelatin. Capsules with a natural filling and coatings are safe, however.

The vitamin B group

The B vitamins are important during illness and recovery, and in general health maintenance. They help to metabolise food, relieve stress and produce antibodies and red blood cells. Chemotherapy and radiotherapy patients need three times the usual amount – during treatment and for two weeks afterwards take 100mg daily each of vitamin B1 (thiamine) and vitamin B6, as well as a general vitamin B complex tablet. All B vitamins are water-soluble and cannot be stored in the body and so a daily intake is essential. These vitamins tend to work together, and so are best take in a balanced formula: an excess intake of any one B vitamin will upset the balance of the group as a whole. The vitamins are vulnerable to alcohol, sugar, some antibiotics and the contraceptive pill.

Natural food sources include fresh green vegetables. Avoid brewer's yeast as a source of vitamin B, as many therapists believe that brewer's yeast is not good for cancer patients and it can also aggravate thrush (Candida albicans).

There is some disagreement about whether cancer patients should take vitamin B12. It could be in short supply if you are on a mostly fruit and vegetable diet, but some therapists believe that it can be a tumour growth-enhancer if taken in excess. Get advice on the dosage and taken an 'enteric coated' tablet, which will prevent the B12 vitamin from being destroyed by stomach acids before it is digested.

Folic Acid is a B vitamin that is important in the synthesis of nucleic acids. Its role is interdependent with that of vitamin B12, and a deficiency of one may lead to a deficiency in the other. A deficiency in folic acid can lead to anaemia. It has a role to play as an anti-oxidant for the health of the blood, glands and liver, and supports the immune system. It is found in leafy green vegetables, bananas and citrus fruit, but if taken in supplement form, take a dosage of 100 microgrammes a day.

Vitamin E

Vitamin E helps prevent the formation in the body of 'free radicals', those over-active atomic particles which damage the genetic structure of cells. It also strengthens the lining of blood vessels and acts as an anti-coagulant. Where cancer is concerned, it can block the formation of carcinogens like nitrosamines, or prevent carcinogens from taking an active form. The *New England Journal of Medicine* reported that hair loss was less common among chemotherapy patients taking vitamin E.

Like vitamins A and C, it stimulates the immune system, and may be able to revert new cancer cells back to normal ones. Vitamin E can be found in vegetable oils, wheatgerm, eggs, fish, nuts, wholegrains, leafy vegetables and cereals. It is difficult to suffer a deficiency, but female cancer patients should tread warily with this vitamin, as it is often linked with the reproductive process and hormone activity (see p.68).

However, the Bristol Cancer Help Centre believes that vitamin E's anti-cancer functions outweigh any effect it may have on hormonal functioning. If you are taking supplementary capsules, take only 100 iu of vitamin E every two days.

MINERALS

Vitamins need minerals in order to perform. Minerals are part of our bones, teeth, soft tissue muscle, blood and nerve cells. The body doesn't produce any minerals, so we must get them from our diet. A cancer patient should take supplements of certain minerals (see below) to make sure that she is getting enough.

Minerals are bound up with different molecules, because they are difficult to digest in a natural form. For instance, in zinc 'picolinate' the mineral zinc is bound to picolinic acid. Minerals bind well to the following binding molecules: picolinates, citrates, aspartates and ascorbates. There are others, but they are harder for the body to assimilate, (for instance, sulphates and oxides).

Zinc, potassium and magnesium

Zinc, potassium and magnesium are needed by a number of enzymes which help to protect the immune system, and although they are best obtained from food, they could be lacking in a Western diet as a result of modern farming methods.

Zinc is a trace element used in the metabolism of food, which helps certain enzymes in tissue healing and regeneration. The immune system needs zinc to function properly. A deficiency could lead to retarded growth in the sex organs. One sure sign of a zinc deficiency is horizontal white specks on the fingernails; other signs are lethargy, and loss of the sense of taste. Zinc is found in herring, wheatgerm, eggs, wholemeal bread, carrots, sweetcorn, non-fat (skimmed) milk powder and mustard. Zinc is thought by herbalists to be good for those cancers that ulcerate, like breast cancer. Take 50 mg of zinc citrate daily – this provides 15 mg of zinc – as the other zinc salts can cause diarrhoea.

Potassium in the body's cells is always in a delicate balance with sodium (salt) in the surrounding tissues. A deficiency of potassium means that sodium can enter the cells and interfere with cell functioning. The balance between sodium and potassium can be maintained by eating a healthy diet and cutting down on processed foods which tend to contain added salt. Potassium helps with muscle tone. Good sources are citrus fruits, watercress, bananas, avocados, apples, grapes, green-leafed vegetables, nuts and potatoes in their skins. If you contract diarrhoea as a result of radiotherapy or chemotherapy, potassium can help – take 600 mg of potassium aspartate daily until the symptoms clear. Otherwise, take 200 mg daily.

Magnesium along with potassium, pushes any excess sodium out of the cells that is interfering with their function. Low magnesium levels, like low selenium levels, seem to correspond with an increased cancer incidence in the general population. Where levels are high in the soil, the cancer incidence is low – but the use of nitrates in agricultural fertiliser locks magnesium in the soil. Magnesium is also required as a helper in producing approximately ninety enzymes, and is needed for the proper functioning of muscle and nervous tissue. Processing destroys magnesium in white bread, white rice and canned or frozen vegetables, but you can find it in fresh green leafy vegetables, fish, meat, nuts, poultry, bran, honey, brewer's yeast and wholemeal flour. The general anti-cancer diet (see p.186) should provide enough magnesium, but you can take a supplement of up to 500 mg twice a day, preferably as an ascorbate or an aspertate.

Magnesium needs calcium in order to be absorbed in the body – you can get the right balance in foods like molasses, bananas, nuts and seeds; or take a supplement of magnesium with calcium in the form of an aspartate so that they balance each other.

Selenium is a trace element needed in small amounts; it is usually found in the soil and taken up by vegetables, but the amount in the soil varies from country to country, and from one part of a country to another. It appears to be a cancer preventative – when it is high in the soil, as in north Norfolk, there is a low incidence of cancer. Some studies have linked a decrease in the soil to an increase in breast cancer. It has a blocking action on tumour-causing agents, and stimulates the immune system into killing new cancer cells. It is also an anti-oxidant.

You can find selenium in free-range poultry, wholegrains, wheatgerm, brewer's yeast, eggs, liver, asparagus, garlic, nuts, fish and seaweed. As it is difficult to tell whether or not it is in your food, you could take it as a supplement. The maximum daily does is 200 micrograms, as large doses are toxic. Selenium toxicity shows up in the ridging and breaking of fingernails, so reduce the dosage if this occurs. The ANAC recommends that selenium should be taken in its organic form, and not as a 'selenite' (a 'salt' form of selenium). The 'selenate' form is OK, and 'L-seleno methionine' is considered by one biologist to be the best form. Selenium is especially useful to take alongside vitamin C, as together they make a good anti-oxidant mix.

ENZYMES

Enzymes are natural substances that either start or contribute to important functions in the body. One of their jobs is to break food down into simpler substances for better absorption. Proteolytic enzymes, which are digestive enzymes that cause the breakdown of protein, have the ability to stimulate the immune system, digest weak cells and prevent the spread of cancer cells. Some enzymes are produced in the body, but the most biologically active enzymes are those of vegetable origin, and raw vegetables are full of them – the cooking process kills enzymes.

Some therapists believe that enzymes hold the highest possibility for the treatment of all cancers: the German cancer therapist's Drs. Hans Nieper and Josef Issels have used enzymes successfully in combination with other techniques. Although there is no scientific evidence in yet, enzymes are thought to strip cancer cells of their protective coatings, so that the immune system can recognise and attack them.

One of the enzymes' strongest roles is in destroying 'free radicals', those supercharged molecules which are unstable due to the loss of an electron, and which try to regain their missing electron from other cells, thus disrupting them. Free radicals are highly reactive cellular toxins that can cause extensive damage on a cellular level throughout the body. Many scientists believe that free radical damage is the precursor to such chronic diseases as cancer, arthritis, heart disease, multiple sclerosis, diabetes and a range of allergic and inflammatory conditions. Normally, free radicals are neutralised by the production of specific enzymes (called 'anti-oxident enzyme complexes') by the cells, but environmental pollutants and exposure to ultraviolet radiation have increased excess free radicals, while lapses in a healthy diet can reduce the body's ability to produce enough protective enzymes. These are the enzymes that devour free radicals:

Super-oxide dismutase – a potent anti-oxident enzyme which changes free radicals into hydrogen peroxide for other enzymes like catalase to deal with.

Catalase is one of the body's strongest, naturally occurring free radical scavenging enzymes, which rids the body of unbalanced oxygen in the form of the 'superoxide' free radical.

Co-enzyme Q10 has been shown to be beneficial in life-extension experiments, and it plays an essential role in the body by helping to release energy from food to feed the cells.

Glutathione peroxidase (GP) removes the free radicals called 'lipid peroxides', which attack the lipid (fat) content of cell membranes.

Methione reductase (MR) is the only enzyme that removes the hydrozyl radical, which is created by exposure to various types of radiation such as the sun, X-rays and cosmic radiation. It is a critical enzyme, because the body cannot make it, and it can be found in grains, fruits and vegetables.

These enzymes can be taken as supplements, in the form of tablets which are made from selectively bred wheat sprouts. The sprouts are one of the richest sources of enzymes. They are available from Nutritec, a company specialising in natural diet supplements (see the list of addresses on p.287).

There are claims that a special blood test (the Le Garde Test), developed in Germany some years ago, can actually show improvement in the blood of arthritics, cancer patients and asthmatics within forty-eight hours of taking large doses of anti-oxidant enzyme complexes. Large doses are also said to help offset the damage caused to healthy cells by chemotherapy and radiotherapy. For advice on dosage, consult Nutritec or your therapist – but the wheat sprouts are harmless and without side effects so there is no danger of over-dosing.

NATUROPATHY

For specific nutritional advice and guidance you can seek the help of a nutritionist, but as such experts tend to be thin on the ground and have no official organisations representing them, it may be easier to find a naturopath. Naturopaths believe that a healthy diet and lifestyle will prevent disease from starting in the first place, and they aim to get the body back to health by stimulating the elimination of toxins. To this end, you may be put on a fast under supervision, or a diet of mostly raw foods, unrefined carbohydrates and a small amount of protein. Naturopaths also believe that illness is an attempt by the body to get back to normal, so symptoms are never suppressed. In fact, a high temperature is often encouraged, to sweat out the waste products.

Naturopaths usually have a background in osteopathy, chiropractic or Alexander Technique and so can help you with any muscle or bone problems as well as dietary ones. They can give advice on relaxation, exercise, posture and breathing too, and some of them use hydrotherapy (water treatment), which involves the application of hot and cold water in the form of baths, packs and douches.

Naturopathy is a useful adjunct to any other treatment that you undertake, whether orthodox or complementary. Check whether your naturopath is fully qualified or just a part-timer, and ask whether he/she has treated cancer patients before. Look under 'Naturopathy' in the list of addresses (p.276) for contacts.

The NHS can pay

If you are resident in the UK, it *is* possible, as a cancer patient, to obtain your vitamins and minerals and some of the supplements prescribed by your GP on the NHS, although some doctors may not realise this. The Bristol Cancer Help Centre has received written confirmation from the Prescription Pricing Authority in Newcastle-upon-Tyne that these things can be ordered on the NHS and passed for payment by them. So don't be afraid to pass this information on to your GP, as you will save yourself some money.

SUPPLEMENTS

There is a group of various substances used by complementary therapists in the fight against cancer which, for want of a better title, I have labelled 'supplements'. Some of these are mentioned below even though they may not be appropriate or available, because women may have heard of them and should have clearer information about them.

Laetrile

Laetrile, or amygdalin as it is also called, is the most controversial of these supplements. It is derived mainly from apricot kernels, although it can be extracted from the pips/kernals of apples, grapes, peaches, pears, nectarines, plums and cherries too. It is also found in unprocessed buckwheat and millet, chick peas, watercress, beansprouts, nuts, mung beans, blackberries, gooseberries and raspberries. Laetrile has been given a vitamin name, B-17, as it is a 'nitriloside' (a water-soluble food factor found in the seeds of most fruits).

This is the theory on how laetrile works: when the nitriloside, or vitamin B-17, is in the system, an enzyme (beta-glucosidase) from the cancer cell splits the nitriloside molecule into two sugar molecules, one of which is benzaldehyde and the other hydrogen cyanide. Normal cells have a fluid around them called 'rhodanese', which protects them against this naturally occurring cyanide in vitamin B-17, but cancer cells do not and so the cyanide destroys them. In this way, B-17 harms only malignant cells. The benzoldehyde molecule may also be destroying cancer cells, in a combined action with the cyanide – and some Japanese researchers believe that benzaldehyde may be more active then the cyanide. Certain orthodox doctors who have tested laetrile in the USA say that there is no proof that it does this, and that it can actually be dangerous to use. Other doctors and therapists claim that the laetrile used in the trials was not pure, was not used as part of a total anti-cancer programme, and was used on terminal patients only – in other words, the results were slanted towards failure.

As a result of the controversy, laetrile has actually been banned in the USA and UK, although it is used in Mexico, most notably at the clinic of Dr Ernesto Contreras, and at other alternative clinics around the world. Dr Contreras, who is a well-respected doctor specialising in cancer treatment, has used laetrile with varying degrees of success on many of his patients, but the American orthodox medical establishment is not convinced by just case histories. Advocates of laetrile admit that it is best used as a preventative, and must be accompanied by a completely vegetarian diet – and you need quite a lot of pure laetrile in order for it to work, which is expensive. It is not known to have any negative side effects.

One doctor who worked for a time at the Santa Maria Hospital in Mexico saw various cancers respond to laetrile, including cancer of the uterus. At one time the Bristol Cancer Help Centres used to advocate it, but it now says only that it may be useful for some people and that the evidence supporting it is 'anecdotal'. Biologist John Stirling has looked at the chemical make-up of laetrile time and time again, and although he doesn't believe that it can kill cancer cells, he feels that it may be a good free-radical scavenger. Some therapists believe the laetrile can ease the pain of secondary cancers, control nausea and possibly help tumour shrinkage.

There is nothing to stop people from getting laetrile naturally, in the foods that they eat. You could crack open the stones of the fruits mentioned above and eat the kernels *alongside the fruit*, in order to get the right balance of vitamins A and C as well as the vitamin B-17. You could eat up to five kernels, three times a day on an empty stomach, leaving four hours between doses. Prepare the kernels by grinding them to a fine powder, then mixing this with water to form a paste, which should be swallowed without chewing so that the anti-cancer properties are not liberated too soon.

For more information on laetrile, see p.288.

Bromelain

Bromelain is a concentrate of protein-digesting enzymes which is found in pineapple. It is thought to damage the protein covering of cancer cells without hurting normal cells, and also keeps the bloodstream flowing clearly. There is no confirmed evidence about bromelain, although some people have found it helpful. The suggested dosage is 100 mg tablets, taken four times daily before meals.

Gamma-linolenic acid

Gamma-linolenic acid (GLA) is an essential fatty acid found in evening primrose oil, blackcurrants and borage. It is thought to help stimulate the production of prostaglandin E1 (PG E1), which is a hormone-like substance and the first stage of development for the immune cells which protect the genetic structure of the body's cells. Many cancer cells appear to have lost the enzyme that makes GLA, and there is some evidence that GLA can stop cancer cells from multiplying. It has shrunk tumours in rats, but it is still being tested in humans.

Although evening primrose oil is usually the source of GLA that most people are familiar with, it is not the best source. Evening primrose oil is a polyunsaturated oil, which many therapists believe should be restricted in cancer patients. A cheaper and better source of GLA is blackcurrant capsules which are lower in polyunsaturated oil and in which the GLA make-up is similar to that in breast milk. Some GLA products may be available on the NHS. The suggested dose is 500 mg, taken one to three times daily in divided doses.

Ginseng

Although ginseng is a natural source of steroids which protects against stress-related diseases and also helps to raise immunity, it is not recommended for female cancer patients as it is a hormone stimulant (see p.67).

IMMUNOTHERAPY

Immunotherapy involves getting the patient's immune system to recognise that the patient is in a diseased state. This therapy is mostly aimed at raising the body's own defences against cancer, rather than mounting a direct assault against the cancerous cells. Giving cancer antigens back to a patient, for example, switches on the immune system, as there is finally a recognition factor.

Immunotherapy was touched upon on p.43, but it is also used by complementary therapists who have trained first as medical doctors. The principle of injecting the patient with various substances to improve the immune response is the same as in the orthodox approach, but the substances, or 'immuno-stimulants', used by complementary doctors and therapists are much more varied. The immuno-stimulants come from the patient's own body, or from cells cultivated in the laboratory, or from animals or plants, or from other outside sources.

One of the strongest proponents of immunotherapy was Dr Josef Issels, who ran his own clinic in Bavaria – before he retired to California, he had the best track record for cancer remissions, cures and overall survival times. He was independently assessed by three different groups of medical personnel who discovered that fifteen years after treatment, 17 per cent of his *terminal* patients were alive, well and without a trace of cancer in their body. This compares with only a 1 per cent success rate for terminal cancer patients who have had orthodox treatment, and includes all patients who have survived only five years, whether they still have cancer in their body or not. Better still, 80 per cent of those cancer patients who Issels was able to treat early were 'disease-free' fifteen years after his therapy.

Issels believes that cancer is not a localised disease limited to the part of the body where the tumour is, but a disease of the whole body. He treated his patients with vaccines made from the patient's own infected teeth and tonsils or from their intestinal flora, in order to desensitise body cells so that they could function normally. Weakened cancer cells from the patient's own cancer were cultivated and injected back into the patient to create more antibodies. Oxygen and ozone infusions were given to weaken the cancer as the disease does poorly in an oxygen-rich environment.

Issels also used injections of gamma globulin to provide fresh antibodies; injections of spleen extracts from immunised animals to increase the patient's white blood cell count; RNA and DNA injections from various sources to change the messages coming from cancerous cells to more normal ones; and vaccines made from the peptides in blood protein to shrink and control tumours. He also used a technique called 'anti-viral blood irradiation' which involved taking out a small amount of the patient's blood, exposing it to ultraviolet rays and returning it to the patient on a drip, so increasing the anti-viral capacity of the blood.

It sounds like a lot of injections, but not every patient received or needed every immunisation technique.

Most patients, however, were injected with weakened *E. coli* virus to create a fever response, which in turn shakes up the immune system, detoxifies the body and stimulates white blood cell production; and cancer cells do poorly at high temperatures. The treatment is always done in a clinic, so that the patient is kept under constant observation during her fever period. It is interesting to note that creating a fever is something done by orthodox doctors to evoke an immune response in certain cases: the simplest way to do it is to pile blankets on a patient while keeping the patient's head cool with an ice-bag, and watching the temperature rise carefully until it reaches the desired degree.

Penny Brohn, one of the founders of the Bristol Cancer Help Centre, underwent immunotherapy treatment and experienced 'fever times' when she went to Issels's former Ringberg clinic to help her breast cancer. She writes about her experiences there in her book *Gentle Giants*.

Issels always used immunotherapy as part of a broader programme of holistic cancer treatments, which included a vegetarian diet with sprouted grains, large doses of enzymes, certain vitamins (A, B complex, C and E), trace minerals and organ preparations; exercise in the fresh air; meditation and so on. He would also use short bursts of chemotherapy and radiotherapy on a patient if he felt he/she needed it. Issels was the first doctor/oncologist to use doses of chemotherapy beyond those recommended at the time (the 1950s) without losing a patient. He maintained that this was because he used other therapies *alongside* chemotherapy.

It is ironic that Issels began to use immunotherapy over forty years ago, and yet today there are doctors who claim that immunotherapy in some form is one of the most promising aspects of future cancer treatment. Biologist John Stirling, who was cured by Issels of stage 3 malignant melanoma fourteen years ago and who worked alongside him for three years, believes strongly that immunotherapy holds the best prospects of survival for breast, uterine and ovarian cancers, and possibly for all cancers.

Although the kind of immunotherapy treatment that Issels carried out is still being used to some degree in America and Europe by orthodox medical doctors who have broadened their treatment base, it is available in England only in the limited form described on p.43, and only through orthodox trained doctors. It would be dangerous for non-medically trained therapists to treat patients in this way; besides which they would need laboratories and other stringent medical back-up facilities. If you are interested in immunotherapy, it is worth checking with the ANAC and the Bristol Cancer Help Centre to see if they know who is doing this work.

Iscador

One immuno-stimulant being used widely by orthodox doctors and complementary therapists alike, both in England and Europe, is Iscador, or Mistletoe extract. It must always be given by a professional therapist/doctor trained in its use.

Iscador is used to destroy cancer cells and to stimulate the immune system. It was developed by Rudolf Steiner, the Austrian scientist and philosopher who also founded Anthroposophy, which is the understanding of man in all his dimensions – physical, mental, spiritual, scientific and cultural. Although Iscador is considered an anthroposophical medicine, it is also used by homoeopaths, and was suggested by Steiner as a cancer treatment on the basis of his spiritual research. It can be understood along the homoeopathic principle of 'like cures like'.

Mistletoe, like cancer, is a parasite that thrives at the expense of its host. It is unusual in that some aspects of its biochemistry are half-way between those of plant and an animal, and it contains numerous amino acids – one of them arginine, is otherwise found only in fish sperm and the liver of mammals.

To produce Iscador, male and female flowers of the mistletoe are mixed in a special centrifuge and certain substances, such as a specific metallic salt, are added, depending upon what cancer is being treated. The mixing process is quite complicated and can involve mixing the juices of flowers from a summer and a winter harvest.

Iscador has had success with female cancers, especially breast cancer. Mistletoe grows on different trees, and each type has an affinity with a specific cancer: for instance, that found grown on apple trees is mostly used for cancers of the female reproductive organs and of the breast, although a post-menopausal woman with breast cancer will fare better with Mistletoe grown on pine trees.

Iscador has been used for years in Europe and there are many clinical papers to show its beneficial effects on different cancers at their various stages of development. It has both a direct and an indirect effect on a cancer tumour. It is said not only to kill cancer at a cellular level, but also to stimulate an immune reaction at the same level, and to help to sort out the misguided genetic messages for cell growth. As most cancer therapies kill cancer cells but produce toxic side effects to the immune system, Mistletoe therapy could be considered nothing short of revolutionary in its approach!

As far as breast cancer is concerned, there is an enormous variety of outcomes and so it is difficult to obtain enough numbers to verify results, but anthroposophical doctors reckon that the survival rate for breast cancers can be *doubled* across the board. A Swiss study on ovarian cancer patients representing all stages of the disease showed that Iscador used as post-operative treatment, with or without radiotherapy, extended survival time in *all* stages. Iscador does not achieve the same results when taken alongside chemotherapy, however. This is because chemotherapy is an immuno-suppressant and Iscador an immuno-stimulant. But Iscador treatment is beneficial when used before and after chemotherapy.

In patients with inoperable tumours, Iscador has been shown to keep the tumours stable for years, allowing patients to live symptom-free lives without the side effects of chemotherapy. Other results affecting the whole patient include deeper sleep, better appetite, the relief of tension and depression, a reduced need for pain relief and an improvement in general health. Doctors using Iscador often prescribe it prior to surgery, as it helps encapsulate a tumour, making it easier to remove.

Iscador is normally given as a course of seven injections, with three injections given a week. It normally takes two to three weeks to take effect. The *immediate* reaction involves a rise in temperature, stimulation of the thymus gland and an increase in white blood cells and antibodies. The degree of temperature rise is determined by the strength of the preparation. A slight inflammatory reaction may be caused at the site of the injection by the stronger doses, which may result in pain or itching, but this can be avoided by modifying the treatment slightly. The dosage varies with each person – the idea is to increase the dosage strength until there is a 'response'. In this way the individual optimal dose can be found, and this is best done in a residential clinic.

Treatment can be carried on lifelong, but if there has been no recurrence of cancer after many years, treatment may be reduced to two to three short courses annually. Iscador injections can be given on the NHS, so once your maintenance dose has been established by an anthroposophical doctor, a letter can be written to your GP with details as to how to continue the injections. According to anthroposophical doctors, the sooner Iscador treatment is started for a cancer, the better the results.

Case Study – ISCADOR

Katherina Collins is considered to be the longest-surviving breast cancer patient ever to have taken part in treatments at the Bristol Cancer Help Centre.

Katherina was forty when she discovered a pea-sized lump in her left breast – but as her husband was dying of stomach cancer at the time, she kept it to herself. When he eventually died two years later, in 1973, another disaster was to follow: the bailiff arrived and took possession of her house and property for payment of business debts incurred during her husband's long illness. Katherina and her two teenaged sons were rehoused in a one-bedroom council flat, and at this point, when Katherina was at her lowest ebb and didn't care if she lived or died, the lump began to grow rapidly and actually broke through the skin. For the next seven years she watched her cancer grow. (Katherina has a type of breast cancer called 'ductal carcinoma', which is a relatively non-aggressive type, as compared to the more common adenocarcinoma. Luckily it was slow-growing, but no one should wait this long before having a lump checked.)

Eventually, she approached her old friend and GP, Douglas

Latto, who confirmed her own diagnosis of cancer. The extent of the raw wound made Dr Latto recommend a mastectomy – this recommendation was echoed by doctors and specialists in America when Katherina went there to visit her brother. However, she resisted surgery – not only because she had always used natural therapies, but also because she had come to distrust orthodox doctors during her husband's long illness. She also didn't want to be a burden to her sons if she ended up in hospital. Finally, under great pressure from her family while in America, Katherina agreed to have a lumpectomy and a biopsy of the seven lymph nodes nearby. The lump and all the lymph nodes revealed the presence of a malignancy, but scans showed no spread of the cancer. The doctor wanted to perform a radical mastectomy and start radiotherapy and chemotherapy, but Katherina refused and returned to England. Within four weeks her lump had grown back to twice its size. Her legs were also being affected, and she thought it was just a matter of waiting to die.

In view of her rejection of orthodox techniques, Dr Latto suggested she try twice-weekly injections of Iscador. She agreed and has continued with these injections, having them as often as she feels she needs them. She's a firm believer that they make her feel better and it is the only physical treatment she has ever had for her breast cancer.

At the same time as starting Iscador treatment, Katherina discovered the Bristol Cancer Help Centre, and for the next three years she visited the centre weekly. Already a vegetarian, she was keen to explore visualisation, meditation and relaxation (see pp. 245 – 251). She was already familiar with spiritual healing and is a spiritual medium herself. The most important thing imparted to her at Bristol, however, was a sense of her own ability to help herself, a strengthening of a belief in her own power.

In 1983, ten years after her lump was discovered, Dr Latto pronounced Katherina to be 'clinically clear' of cancer: her tumour had by this time shrunk and disappeared. Although her remission/ possible cure may have resulted from a combination of things (the synergistic effect of a positive attitude, healthy diet, visualisation and Iscador, for example), Dr Latto has strong positive feelings about the use of Iscador in particular – based both on the research surrounding it and its effect on his other cancer patients, many of whom have also experienced improved health after taking it.

Research into Iscador

In 1935 the Society for Cancer Research was founded in Arlesheim, Switzerland, by a group of anthroposophical doctors who were working towards the further perfection of Iscador. In 1949 Dr Alexandre Leroi founded the Research Institute, HISCIA, which is dedicated to the manufacture and active promotion of Iscador. A second unit, the WIDAR Research Centre, is involved in chemical and biological studies on Iscador preparations.

Iscador has been well researched in the Lukas clinic in Arlesheim. There are over sixty research papers to date, confirming the positive effects of Mistletoe therapy, and although most of them are in German, some have been translated into English. The case material covers about 7,000 patients, and recently the treatment results for the separate cancers has started to be assessed. To see copies of these clinical trials, write care of The Society for Cancer Research, Kirschweg 9, Ch-4144, Arlesheim, Switzerland.

Iscador is just one type of Mistletoe preparation, but it is the only one licensed for use in Great Britain, which means it can be prescribed by any registered doctor. Other Mistletoe preparations, which are made in Germany, have to be brought into the country on the specific request of a doctor for a patient. These, which have slightly different actions, are used when there is not enough response to Iscador.

You can obtain a list of doctors who will prescribe Iscador from the Anthroposophical Medical Association, c/o Rudolph Steiner House, and The Royal London Homoeopathic Hospital. It is also one of the main cancer treatments given at Park Attwood Clinic, a centre for residental treatment with anthroposophical medicine (conventional and complementary medicine) inspired by Rudolph Steiner. (See the list of addresses on p.276.).

12

Detoxification

Detoxification, or helping the body rid itself of waste products, is thought by many complementary therapists to be important in healing, particularly in the case of cancer. This is because any activity that breaks down tumours will be flooding the bloodstream with toxins from that tumour which need to be removed. This puts a great deal of strain on the liver, the second largest organ of elimination in the body, as well as on the bowels. Drugs and antibiotics make the situation worse by killing off the good bacteria in the gut and allowing the bad bacteria to grow unimpeded.

The colon (large intestine) is an important part of the digestive system: it completes the digestive process and takes care of much of our body's waste products. 1.5m (5 feet) in length and 6 ½ cm (2 ½ inches) in diameter, the colon is divided into three segments: the ascending colon (caecum), which food enters in a fluid state; the transverse colon, where water, vitamins and minerals are re-absorbed; and the descending colon, where mucus coats the faeces to ease passage out of the body. The colon is normally populated by billions of 'friendly' bacteria, which help to detoxify waste and to synthesise certain vitamins. They also play a role in guarding the body against infection. A healthy colon will produce a bowel movement within twenty-four hours of eating, but when illness is present, colon activity can slow down, leading to poor digestion, constipation, diarrhoea or an unhealthy explosion in its yeast population. This can lead to auto-intoxication (self-poisoning), where wastes in the colon are re-absorbed into the bloodstream, so placing a heavy burden on the other eliminative organs of the body: the kidneys, skin and lungs. It is clear, therefore that the proper functioning of the colon is necessary for good health.

It could be said that certain diets, vitamins, herbs and various supplements detoxify the body in a *wider* sense. Detoxification can also mean special baths of herbs, Epsom salts or ozone which help the skin, the largest organ of elimination, to flush out toxins through the pores. But detoxification for the cancer patient mainly means coffee enemas and colonic cleansing. Neither of these techniques, however, may be suitable for a female cancer that has spread to the abdomen, or where there is rectal bleeding or trouble in passing stools suggesting a blockage, so take advice first from your doctor and therapist. Seeking advice about coffee enemas is particularly relevant for people with cardiovascular disease, as the enema may produce symptoms of tachycardia (when the heart beats faster than normal).

COFFEE ENEMAS

Coffee enemas are used a great deal in Europe and the USA for liver stimulation. The Gerson Diet (see p.194) uses them as an integral part of its strategy – while the juices and foods of the almost entirely vegan diet stimulate tumour breakdown, the coffee enema stimulates the liver to remove toxins, and stimulates peristaltic wave movements of the colon. It also causes the gall bladder to flush out bile and toxins, which in turn revitalises the liver.

The idea of giving yourself an enema may make many women very squeamish, but I have been assured by advocates of the technique that once you have tried it, and experienced how much better you feel afterwards, it quickly becomes part of your daily routine for regaining your health. It also helps to give relief from pain. An enema means taking in liquid through the rectum and holding it for as long as you can. The idea is to work with up to 600ml (1 pint) of coffee. The coffee is absorbed into the bloodstream through the veins in the rectum and reaches the liver through the portal vein. Once in the liver, the coffee stimulates the production of bile, which carries waste products out of the body.

All that you need is a gravity-fed enema kit which you can buy from some chemists. You can use tinned or freshly ground coffee (organic preferably), but not instant coffee, which has added chemicals. If you are weak, you may need someone to help you. The best description of a coffee enema is given by Brenda Kidman in her book, *A Gentle Way With Cancer*; here is an abridged version:

1. First, make the coffee: put 1 – 3 tablespoons of tinned ground or freshly ground coffee into 1.2 litres (2 pints) of water and boil for three minutes. Turn down the head and simmer for fifteen minutes, then cool and strain. The coffee should be at body temperature for the enema.

2. Fit up the enema kit in the bathroom, so that the container is hanging at least 60cm (2 feet) above where you are lying. Put a pillow and a piece of plastic sheeting or an old towel on the floor to lie on. Take a book or the radio for company as the whole procedure takes twenty minutes.

3. After closing the tap on the enema tube, poor 600ml (1 pint) of blood-heat coffee into the container.

4. Release the tap and allow some coffee to flow out, preferably into the empty container that the coffee was brought in, to ensure that all the air is out of the tube.

5. Turn off the tap, then pour the coffee back into the enema container.

6. Grease the nozzle of the catheter with KY Jelly. Lying on your side with your knees up and consciously relaxing, push the catheter gently into the rectum. This is not as difficult as it sounds, and it is not painful. If you 'bear down' as you push in the catheter, it will help to widen the rectal opening.

7. With the catheter in place, turn on the tap until you feel the coffee flowing in. Let it flow in slowly, and when all the coffee has passed in, turn off the tap and remove the catheter.

8. Massage your stomach to help the enema to be spread through your colon, and relax for fifteen minutes. Then go to the lavatory to let the enema pass out.

COLONIC CLEANSING

Colonic cleansing (also known as colonic irrigation, colon hydrotherapy, or simply as a colonic) was first recorded in Ancient Egypt in 1500 BC. It can be described as an internal bath that helps to cleanse the colon of poisons, gases and any accumulation of mucus or faeces. Basically, filtered water is gently introduced into the rectum through sterilised equipment to soften and help expel any compacted deposits. Colonic cleansing differs from an enema in that water is not retained in the rectum; instead, clean water passes in and dirty water passes out in an ebb-and-flow movement. It is not something that you can do for yourself; a competent colonic therapist must do it for you.

The technique helps to move along wastes that have become trapped in the colon due to sluggish bowel movements. The bowel can become sluggish as a result of poor diet, radiotherapy, chemotherapy or the cancer itself. Because of the decrease in the natural wave-like action of the bowel there is a build-up of toxins in the system, which can damage the colon and re-enter the bloodstream. This in turn lowers the body's immune defences even further.

Treatment with colonics is not a 'cure all' for cancer; rather, its strongest role is as a cancer preventative. It is best used alongside other therapies, such as special diet, herbalism and homoeopathy, and can actually enhance their action. Apart from toxin removal it can offer increased vitality, pain relief and a feeling of well-being. Colonics cannot be used by any cancer patients with abdominal obstruction, severe anaemia, severe haemorrhoids, gastro-intestinal haemorrhage or perforation, weak kidneys or cancer of the colon, or by anyone who has had recent colon surgery.

How the treatment is given

During the treatment the patient, wearing a hospital gown and covered by a blanket, lies on her back on a table. A speculum (tube) is gently inserted into the rectum. This tube has two branches: one for the passage of clean filtered water into the colon, and the other through which dirty water and waste can pass out. The water temperature, pressure and flow time are carefully controlled by the therapist, and water is progressively fed around the colon. A viewing window in the machine allows the therapist to see what is being eliminated. The British manufacturers of one machine plan to add a computer print-out which will instantly analyse what passes out.

The tube may be either disposable or non-disposable, depending on the machine used. The non-disposable type is sterilised between use in a powerful hospital antiseptic called Sporicidin,which is strong enough to kill even the Aids virus.

After the colon has been filled up, the therapist helps the movement of water around the colon by gently massaging the patient's abdomen. After most of the water has been expelled, more water is circulated through. An average colonic takes half an hour – any longer tends to exhaust the colon. Most often a six-week course is recommended, with one treatment a week, but this can vary and depends on what agreement you have reached with your therapist. Colonics are not normally given more than twice a week, except when a patient is resident in the hospital or clinic, allowing extra care to be taken of her. Contrary to popular belief, colonics with pure filtered water do not remove essential electrolyte minerals from the body: blood tests have proved this.

Various substances can be added to the inflowing water, depending on the patient's condition: for instance, oxygen, which acts as a natural antibiotic and kills thrush (*Candida albicans*) and other anaerobic (oxygen-hating) parasites; aloe vera, to regulate and soothe the digestive tract; or a high concentration of broad-spectrum bacilli to restore 'friendly' bacteria. Other additions include Epsom salts, fennel and camomile tea. Vitamin and mineral drinks are sometimes given to the patient after treatment to counteract any tendency towards fatigue, and probiotics are given orally to boost the 'friendly' bacteria count (see p. 223).

There is no discomfort in the treatment – in fact, in a setting which often includes soft music and a pastel-coloured treatment room, the temptation is to fall asleep! If the patient is very toxic, or if the water hits a pocket of gas, there might be a slight colicky pain, but this is easily relieved by abdominal breathing and massage. Although patients usually feel good after a colonic, side effects can include gas, colicky pains, headache, nausea and light-headedness, but this simply indicates that the body is continuing to remove toxins effectively.

The main benefit is rapid detoxification. Other benefits for cancer patients include relief from the pain and discomfort of any gastro-intestinal problems as well as from skin irritations, fatigue, cold hands and feet and mild haemorrhoids.

Used as a preventative, a colonic can remove encrusted toxins, thus reducing the strain on the liver and kidneys, and stimulate the colon to regain its natural shape and tone. It can also help to prevent colon cancer, the second most common type of cancer. Even those in good health can benefit from a colonic: athletes and singers, for example, are amazed at how much more lung capacity is created by the removal of toxins. The youngest person to have received a colonic so far is six months old; the oldest is over ninety.

The colonic machines are also equipped to give an enema, which may precede a colonic if hardened waste is difficult to remove. Dr Milo Siewert, president of the Colonic International Association and who runs the Bournemouth Centre for Complementary Medicine (BCCM) uses many different types of herbal enemas: Cayenne to stimulate the liver, kidneys, spleen and pancreas; Garlic or mineral water for general cleansing; Catnip for colic; and Wild Yam and Nettle for gas. But the most common enema is the ground coffee enema (see p.219) which he encourages patients to use at home, not only for liver detoxification, but also because the caffeine stimulates the peristaltic muscle to contract more powerfully and loosen deposits on the colon walls.

It is extremely important for anyone receiving a colonic to supplement their diet with *Lactobacillus acidophilus* to restore the normal balance of bowel flora. As one well-known therapist has said, 'No one with healthy gastro-intestinal bacteria has yet to be found with chronic disease.' Eating live yoghurt is *not* effective, because the number of live bacteria in yoghurt is minimal. Your therapist should be able to recommend or to give to you a supply of active, freeze-dried *Lactobacillus acidophilus* which will contain billions of live organisms per teaspoon! This product must be taken on an empty stomach so that the potency is not destroyed by digestive enzymes. There are *acidophilus* products available for those patients who are sensitive to dairy products as well. The ideal *acidophilus* product also contains a 'friendly' bacteria called *ifidobacterium*; both bacteria work to keep harmful bacteria to a minimum. However, anyone with a weakened immune system should avoid probiotics with *Streptococcus faecium* or *Strephococcus faecilis*, because there is concern that these two organisms are potentially pathogenic

D'Anne Coburn, colonic therapist, has treated women cancer patients. She always takes blood pressure and a urine sample before starting a colonic: if these are not satisfactory, she may not proceed. During treatment she also keeps a close eye on the patient's pulse. D'Anne treats her patients holistically – they may be put on a cleansing diet of organic vegetables and juices during the series of treatments, and a lemon enema which draws out toxins might be given before a colonic. She talks to her patients about their lifestyle and way of thinking – she believes that mental attitude is as important as diet, and she recommends visualisation and relaxation. A patient with breast cancer might also be treated with packs of herbs on the breast which act like a poultice on the cancer by drawing it out.

A woman with an early cancer and strong 'life force', would be given a slow detoxification over two years; a middle-stage cancer would require a faster detoxification; while an advanced cancer patient would still benefit from the treatment in terms of vitality and pain relief. Unfortunately, D'Anne says, cancer patients tend to show up in the late stages of cancer. She believes strongly in using colonics as a *preventative* to cancer: 'If your system is dirty through trauma and stress and not enough oxygen, cell changes will occur. If you can clear up a person's system before the cells change, then you can prevent cancer,' In all cases of cancer she believes that the system is 'congested'; and she looks to the bowel initially for the cause of most disease. She adds, 'If the bowel is blocked up, the circulation and the immune system will be sluggish.'

Case Study – COLONICS

Nicky Ireland was twenty-four when her cervical smear was diagnosed as advanced CIN (the next stage was cervical cancer itself). After laser surgery, Nicky's smear regressed to between CIN 1 and CIN 2, but she was experiencing heavy, painful periods with backaches and headaches. Six months later she underwent a second laser operation, and a D and C (dilatation and curretage) to help with her periods.

At this point Nicky decided to do something to help herself and visited a therapist on a friend's recommendation. The therapist reviewed Nicky's dietary history – which included eating the wrong foods and binges with laxatives to help lose weight – and decided to put her on a series of colonics for detoxification. Nicky had twelve colonics in all, and began to feel much better after the second. By the end of the series her backaches and headaches had completely disappeared.

After the colonics Nicky was given acidophilus to replace the good intestinal flora that had been washed away by the treatment. She was also placed on an 'allergy-free' diet for a time and given high-potency vitamins and minerals to match her dietary needs. Although Nicky was also given homoeopathic drops and 'Rife Light' treatment (pulsed light emitted at a frequency that is harmful to viruses and aberrant cells), she feels strongly that the colonics and diet changes led the way to improvement. 'I feel so much better in myself,' she says, 'and my periods are now lighter, with very little pre-menstrual tension. I'm also more in touch with my body and more aware of which foods disagree with me.'

Two months after beginning her complementary therapy, Nicky's smear was 'clear' and it has remained so. The specialist saw no scar tissue and announced that it 'looked like a different cervix'. Although Nicky used a combination of orthodox and complementary methods to tackle her CIN, she feels that the colonics went a long way towards clearing out her system of accumulated toxins, eased her period problems and made her feel 'clean, both inside and out'.

How to find a colonic therapist

If you want to call on the services of a colonic therapist, find one who has trained with either the Colonics International Association or the International Colonic Hydrotherapy Foundation (see p.284). A good therapist must be a good diagnostician too, to discover problems that the patient may not have known she had. Effective treatment is not defined by the quantity of faeces eliminated but by the therapist's ability to get water into colonic pockets where accumulated toxins lie.

13

Herbalism, Homoeopathy, Acupuncture and Chinese Herbal Medicine

Herbalism, homoeopathy and acupuncture should all be taken as complementary therapies alongside orthodox treatments. As all three of them treat the patient holistically, it is necessary to try only one at a time. If you use more than one of the three together, you won't know what is working, and you will over-stimulate the body.

HERBALISM

Plants have been used medicinally for thousands of years. In fact, a number of medical drugs are derived from herbs: for example, digitalis from the foxglove, morphine from the opium poppy, and aspirin from the willow bark. The theory behind herbalism is that if one part of the body is not functioning properly, further imbalances are created in other parts, with the possibility of illness. Human health can be affected equally by emotional and spiritual problems, as well as by environment and lifestyle. Disease is the result of the body's attempts to restore balance and harmony. In the same way as homoeo-pathy, herbalism supports the body's healing mechanism rather than repressing it.

The herbalist treats the person as a whole entity: there are no separately defined illnesses. An individual picture is made up of each patient, so that what is appropriate treatment for one won't be for another, even with the same illness. The aim of treatment is to assist the body's own healing and return the patient to balanced health. Modern medical herbalists combine traditional knowledge with four years of clinical training based on modern research into pharmacology; they need to know which part of a herb to use, how to prepare it and the correct dosage to give. Herbalists use extracts from the *whole* plant, which is actually safer and has fewer side effects than if isolated plant ingredients are used. Herbs provided in this way cause no imbalances in the body, and also contain vitamins and trace elements.

Herbalists look for the basic cause of an ailment, whether it be infection, injury or stress, and make a detailed 'symptom' picture. Any history of inherited disorders or weaknesses is noted, and a patient is examined in a conventional way, with some conventional medical instruments – for instance, blood pressure is measured conventionally. The first visit takes an hour.

The organs of elimination and the circulatory system are both considered to be important to good health. Symptoms are pushed in the direction that they want to go, so a cough would be encouraged in order to loosen phlegm. If the herbalist feels that stress is a contributory factor relevant in causing the illness, he/she will offer advice on relaxation technique; if the diet is not what it should be, dietary advice will be given, and possible allergies will be discussed. Each person is seen to have a responsibility towards his/her own health, and self-help measures will be suggested to correct any underlying trends that could provoke further ill health.

Prescribed herbal remedies work slowly and gently with no side effects, although they can create permanent effects. There have been few clinical trials on herbs and herbal products, however; claims of success are based on their traditional use over centuries.

Herbal medicine is most often prescribed in the form of a tincture, which is made by 'macerating' the roots, leaves and sometimes the flowers of a herb (removing the soft parts by steeping), and then leaving them to set in a solution of alcohol and water. Alcohol is used because it extracts the maximum of compounds from the plants and also acts as a preservative. Herbal tisanes (dried herbs used for teas) can also be prescribed, or the herbal remedy may come as a syrup, tablets, capsules, lotion, gargle, cream or ointment. Herbal remedies can be classified as stimulants, relaxants and nervous 'restoratives' – this last remedy restores normal nervous functioning after a period of stress or chronic debility.

The dosage is normally three times daily. How quickly you respond depends on how long you have had the problem. With cancer, visits to the herbalist would probably continue as long as the disease was present. Prescriptions will alter according to how your symptoms change.

Herbalism is not a guaranteed cure for cancer, but some cancer tumours have been inhibited by herbal treatment. In fact, many of orthodox medicine's strongest cytotoxic drugs are made from herbs, such as vinblastine. Herbs work in many different ways. Those that help by detoxifying the liver, known as 'alteratives', include Blue Flag, Burdock Root, Yellow Dock, Barberry Bark, Fringe Tea Bark, Dandelion Root, Gentian Root and the leaves from the Century Herb and the Holy Thistle. Burdock Root and Yellow Dock are particularly powerful. The kidneys are helped by Cleavers (Goosegrass) and Dandelion Root. Those herbs that have a toning and cleansing effect on the lymphatic system include Cleavers, Echinacea Root, Poke Root, and Wild Violet Leaves.

Tom Bartram, a herbalist who has practised for many years and is now retired, singles out Poke Root as being anti-bacterial and anti-viral as well as having an effect on tumours, while Wild Violet Leaves seem to help inhibit the spread of cancer. Although no one herb can be used as an antidote for any one cancer, and herbal medicine is prescribed for the total sum of symptoms, the following herbs have been used with varying degrees of success to treat women's cancers: Poke Root for ovarian cancer; Mistletoe, Red Clover, Plantain and Cleavers for uterine and cervical cancers; and Red Clover and Poplar Mistletoe for breast cancer, although Red Clover is not used when there is breast ulceration.

Bartram has seen these herbs cure stages 1 and 2 of the respective female cancers when no other treatment was taken, and even some stage 3s – although many herbalists believe that it is still best to take complementary and orthodox treatments alongside each other. He believes that these herbs are best taken as teas, for then they travel through the system more quickly. To make a herbal tea, use two teaspoons of dried herbs to a cup of boiling water and infuse for fifteen minutes. Take three or more times daily to feel the benefit. Mistletoe, which is normally injected just under the skin in the form of Iscador (see p.213), can be made into a tea by soaking it in cold water overnight.

If you are able to get hold of the whole plant, which consists of the bark, roots and leaves of a herb, the best way to use it, according to Brenda Kidman in her book, *A Gentle Way With Cancer*, is to bring 50g (2oz) of the bark and roots to the boil in 900ml (1 ½ pints) of water and simmer for twenty minutes. Put 25g (1oz) of leaves in a vacuum flask and strain the boiling extract of the bark and roots on to them. Seal the flask, leave overnight and then strain, cool and refrigerate. Take 25ml (1 fl oz) twice daily, diluted if preferred.

To save yourself all this trouble, you could use the liquid extracts of the herbs, although they may not be as fresh or as potent. Brenda Kidman says that if you use the liquid extracts, you can avoid coffee enemas (see p.219)!

According to Dr Jan De Vries, Butterbur (*Petasites officinales*) is a herb which acts as a cell renewer, and it has an influence on swellings and tumours. He claims that breast fibroids have been reduced by concentrated Butterbur extract, but he does not know which substance in the plant or the root is the active ingredient. Butterbur has been used since early Roman times.

More recently on the scene is Lapacho (Ipe Roxo), also known as Pau d'Arco. Lapacho is a South American tree whose bark can be made into a tea or tonic. Research is still continuing on this herb, but it appears to be good at breaking up tumours, and has been used with some success in treating leukaemia.

Herbalists believe that healing comes only from the body's own innate 'healing force' and that herbs can help this. Because the herbal compounds are so complex, they must always be obtained from a qualified practitioner (see p.287). Self-medication should never be attempted, especially with herbs that you have picked yourself, as some are toxic – in fact, the dosages of some herbal medicines are strictly controlled by law. We all know about Deadly Nightshade (*Atropa belladonna*), but were you aware that too much Sage could cause a miscarriage, or too much Comfrey a liver tumour? Also, some herbs can absorb heavy metals: for example, Dandelion and Horsetail can pick up mercury. And if you buy off-the-shelf remedies, you won't know if the medicine has the correct herbs in the right quantities, or if the product will stay stable over its advertised shelf life.

If a patient in an acute condition approaches a herbalist, she would be referred back or on to a GP or a hospital. Unfortunately, most cancer patients visit herbalists when their disease *is* in an advanced state, as a last-ditch effort after all the orthodox treatments have been exhausted. As one herbalist puts it, 'Cancer patients must put their whole backs into herbal treatment, and do it wholeheartedly. Some patients *do* get over their cancers, with the help of luck, genetics or a lack of stress – but for a rampaging cancer, there may be no cure wherever you go.'

HOMOEOPATHY

Homoeopathy was developed by a German doctor, Samuel Hahnemann, in the nineteenth century. After many years of research, Hahnemann concluded that symptoms were the body's way of attempting to cure itself of illness, and that remedies often caused an intensification of the existing symptoms or a return of old symptoms before the patient began to feel better.

He deduced that any drug which can cause the symptoms of a disease can also *cure* that disease, which led him to devise the underlying homoeopathic principle of 'like cures like'. He also discovered, when faced with the drastic side effects of most of the drugs he was using, that minute doses would work just as well as larger ones; and this became another underlying principle of homoeopathy. He developed a potency scale where remedies were diluted up to many thousands of times, but vigorously shaken between dilutions: strangely enough, increasing the dilution increased the potency of a medicine in a way that is still not fully understood today, but which may have something to do with the energy field of the homoeopathic remedy being left behind.

One scientific explanation for the potency increase is that the transmission of the biological information is somehow related to the molecular organisation of water and the effects of magnetic fields – it has been suggested that magnetic fields affect and restructure the water molecules. The medicine, in effect, leaves behind its molecular 'imprint' on the water, which appears to have stronger effects than the medicine itself. Homoeopathy, then, deals with *energy* that catalyses the body into healing itself.

Hahnemann first tried out all his remedies on healthy people in safe doses to discover what the symptoms would be. These people recorded the effects the drugs were having on them, including not only the physical but also the emotional and mental changes that took place. Today the system works in reverse: a person's physical, emotional and mental symptoms are matched to a specific homoeopathic remedy. Thus the energy in the body is matched to the energy in the remedy. In fact, homoeopaths deny any distinction between physical and mental symptoms: every physical illness has a mental aspect, and every mental illness has a physical aspect.

Homoeopathic treatment aims to eliminate the cause of a disease and not just the symptoms. It doesn't suppress symptoms but pushes the body in the direction that it wants to go: for example, if a person has an infected throat, it may get a little worse after the remedy is given before clearing up. In other words, the remedies enhance the body's natural reactions – such as vomiting in response to food poisoning – in order to rid itself of toxins.

There are many hundreds of homoeopathic remedies and all are chosen specifically for the individual. The choice of a remedy depends on the total symptom picture, but the homoeopath's skill is to discern the most important symptoms that are central to the case. Each individual will have a slightly different experience of an illness depending on her own inherited susceptibilities and her environment. The energy behind a person's symptoms is the body's 'vital' or 'life' force, which is beyond any organ or organ system, being the very breath of life itself. The life force is dynamic and ever-changing, continually reacting and adjusting to internal and external stimuli.

Homoeopathic remedies can treat acute conditions like colds or flu, or chronic illnesses which have lasted for years and which homoeopaths believe can be passed on through the generations of a family. As one homoeopath explained it, remedies can assure that you will reach, over a period of time, an optimum state of health. Simplistically put, it is like peeling off the layers of an onion: as one set of symptoms is cleared up, anything else that arises is then dealt with. Orthodox medicine, on the other hand, suppresses certain symptoms: for example, cytotoxic drugs given for cancer lower the already depleted immune system. The remedies actually change the body's susceptibility to an affliction at a very subtle, possibly a genetic, level. An increase in energy is the first sign that the remedies are working on a deeper level.

HOMOEOPATHY AND CANCER TREATMENT

So where does homoeopathy fit into cancer treatment? Homoeopathic remedies act as catalysts for the body to heal itself, and so can be used to treat all of the female cancers. Some homoeopaths claim to have cured cancer through their methods alone, while others argue that homoeopathy has only a secondary role to play and that it shouldn't interfere with any orthodox treatment, especially surgery. Homoeopathic remedies can be taken alongside orthodox treatments, as they counter the side effects of the drugs and radiotherapy used by helping to increase the strength of the immune system. The side effects of chemotherapy and radiotherapy such as nausea, mouth ulcers, resultant weakness, depression and so on are alleviated by homoeopathic treatment.

Homoeopathy is most helpful in early-stage cancer and pre-cancerous states, and on those patients who have not yet had chemotherapy or radiotherapy. Women who might benefit greatly from homoeopathy are those diagnosed as having CIN, who may often have to wait months between diagnosis and treatment on a long NHS waiting list. Homoeopaths could treat women during that interval – and without other treatments being used alongside it, the benefits of homoeopathy would be more apparent. Also, women with breast lumps, whether benign or malignant, appear to react favourably to homoeopathic treatment.

Many patients don't visit a homoeopath until they are in a late stage of cancer – at this point, the body's 'vital energy' may be just too depleted to bounce back. But homoeopathy can still be of use by relieving symptoms and helping with any pain.

Remedies can be given to help shrink tumours, but the overall state of the patient is taken into account and treated simultaneously, which helps to reduce the susceptibility to cancer and to raise the immune system. Physical improvement would depend on the stage of the cancer. The *internal* physical condition of the organs would need to be verified by orthodox medical techniques. The results to expect from homoeopathy would be increased energy levels, a reduction in anxiety, more optimism and better sleeping patterns. This is particularly noticeable if you take a homoeopathic remedy during or after chemotherapy treatment.

Remedies are made from natural substances such as herbs, salts, minerals and even diseased tissue. Although it is impossible to state which homoeopathic remedy will cure which cancer, because each is prescribed individually, some examples of remedies can be given.

Remedies and their prescription

A remedy called 'Lycopodium' can be used to treat ovarian cysts or breast tumours, as the remedy is effective against different types of growth. '*Asterias rubens*', or 'Red Starfish', is noted for its tumour-shrinking abilities, particularly in breast cancer. A lump in the breast might be treated with Conium (Hemlock), especially if there was a history of grief prior to the appearance of the lump, as Conium is one of the many remedies associated with grief and breast lumps together. Remedies such as Nitric Acid and Phosphoric Acid are both useful in treating chemotherapy-induced side effects. But again, remedies are prescribed only on the basis of the total symptom picture: all the physical, mental and emotional symptoms are taken into consideration in order to find the right prescription.

Homoeopaths are in agreement with recent research in the USA that cancer is often linked with suppressed emotions like anger and grief, usually appearing after a death or a separation. They concur that it is often the emotional level that throws up the susceptibility to cancer when this level is disturbed. But whatever it is that makes the person susceptible, theory has it that it so disturbs the vital force of the body that the body reacts by displaying certain symptoms. These symptoms either resolve themselves or they can form a deeper trauma like a cancer. Although the psyche is important, homoeopaths believe that there can be physical susceptibilities to cancer as well – so that if cancer runs in a family, a woman should seek homoeopathic treatment in order to strengthen her immune system.

Before treating any patient, a homoeopath will gather information about her by asking detailed questions on symptoms, family medical history, events in her emotional life and even reactions to hot and cold. The reason this is done is to look for the *differences* in illnesses: orthodox doctors on the other hand, use a set of common symptoms, and consider the common elements to be more important than the points of difference.

Remedies are usually given first in a single dose in tablet form, dissolved under the tongue. The patient then reports any changes in symptoms over a period of days, weeks or even months. Where a chronic condition is concerned, a single dose may continue to work for months. Normally a treatment begins to work within a range of fifteen minutes to four weeks, depending on the person, the acuteness of the condition and her sensitivity to remedies. Any acute condition is treated first, then the chronic conditions are addressed during subsequent visits to the homoeopath.

A remedy may be repeated, or a different one may be prescribed if there are new symptoms. The subtle art of homoeopathy is prescribing the right remedy, and sometimes several visits are needed before the correct remedy is found.

The beauty of homoeopathic remedies, as practitioners see it, is that they act as catalysts for self-healing, without needing the support of any other approach, such as a special diet. You don't even have to believe in the remedy in order for it to work, although the 'ideal' patient is one who is in touch with her body and notices subtle changes.

PROOF THAT HOMOEOPATHY WORKS

It is difficult to prove how well homoeopathy is working for a female cancer patient who is taking other treatments at the same time which suppress the symptom picture. Homoeopaths can point to their successful case studies, but find it difficult to conduct scientific trials to satisfy the orthodox medical establishment when there are at least twenty or more possible remedies for one disease. At the time of writing, however, clinical trials are being run at the Royal Homoeopathic Hospital in London to test the efficacy of homoeopathic remedies – it is to be hoped that more scientific proof will be forthcoming. The problem is that the empirical method of proof is not applicable to homoeopathic trials, and another model of testing is needed.

Proof that the 'potency theory' works was recently announced in the scientific journal *Nature* after years of research by an international team led by French biologist Professor Jacques Benveniste. The team found that if antibodies were isolated and added to a liquid then diluted until they were no longer present, white blood cells still reacted to the liquid if it was shaken. Homoeopaths claim that this was exactly how their potency theory works – that if a substance is diluted to an ultra-molecular level in a solution, the solution still retains an 'imprint' of the substance if it is vigorously shaken between dilutions.

Benveniste's findings are being disputed in some quarters, and so the debate about *how* homoeopathy works goes on. That it *does* work, however, can be proved by the number of patients who have been successfully treated, and by the fact that it is the second most popular form of complementary medicine after osteopathy.

The future of homoeopathy

The principles of homoeopathy are fast becoming recognised by the work being done in the last few years by certain physicists. There is speculation that one day there will be a machine that can match the energy level of a patient's electro-magnetic field to the electro-magnetic field of a homoeopathic remedy. This may only be a few years away.

How to find a homoeopath

Homoeopathy is the only branch of complementary medicine available on the NHS. Qualified doctors trained in homoeo-pathy can be found by contacting The British Homoeopathic

Association and The Homoeopathic Trust. Non-medically qualified practitioners are to be found by contacting the Society of Homoeopaths (see under 'Homoeopathy' in the list of addresses on p.287). Although not medically qualified, these homoeopaths undergo a long and thorough training over a period of years, which equips them to practise to a very high standard. There are NHS homoeopathic centres in hospitals treating cancer in London, Liverpool, Glasgow, Bristol and Tunbridge Wells. They operate on an outpatient basis, and all you need is a letter from your GP, although there may be long waiting lists.

ACUPUNCTURE AND CHINESE HERBAL MEDICINE

Acupuncture is closest to homoeopathy in the way that it works, because they both work with *energy*. But acupuncture is concerned with balancing different factors in the body. It is used to treat functional disorders, infections and acute or chronic diseases like asthma, migraine or Bell's palsy. Taken alongside orthodox treatments like chemotherapy and radiotherapy, acupuncture can reduce the toxic effects of these treatments and help the blood to recover more quickly, and improve general well-being. It can also ease pain and strengthen the immune system by helping the hormone balance and clearing channels for the circulatory and lymphatic systems. By making adjustments to the energy flow, it can enhance an individual's capacity to heal herself.

Acupuncture *on its own* is not a strong weapon against cancer; combined with Chinese herbs, however it is much more effective for fighting cancer, as the latter are noted for their tumour-fighting abilities. Chinese herbs are quite different from Western herbs and are categorised differently (see p.240).

THE THEORY OF ACUPUNCTURE

Acupuncture derives from ancient Chinese medicine, and traditional Chinese techniques for this method of treatment go back at least 6,000 years. Health is defined as a state of internal harmony, governed by the two principles of 'yin' and 'yang' – disease occurs when the internal harmony is disturbed and the balancing process can no longer cope. Yin represents softness, darkness, coldness and wetness; yang represents hardness, brightness, heat and dryness. The world and the body are defined by these two concepts and you can't have one without the other.

In the body, yin and yang complement each other, with some body parts being more yin and some more yang; in a healthy person they are in a state of constant flux, but also in a state of balance with each other. If there is an imbalance of yin to yang, the body reacts by creating symptoms. An illness has a predominance of yin or yang symptoms. Treatment aims to restore the internal balance.

Another factor concerned in maintaining balance and harmony in the body is the 'five phases': wood, fire, earth, metal and water. Each phase represents a stage in the annual progression of the seasons. In the body the organs, or 'zangfu', and the pathways that link all body parts, the 'jingluo' or 'meridians' (there are twelve of these), each correspond to one of the five phases.

The relationship between the organs is similar to that between the seasons, where each supports the other through their separate but interrelated functions. Some organs are 'zang', meaning they are solid, store 'qi' (see below) and are yin-oriented like the lungs, spleen and heart; other organs are 'fu', meaning they are hollow and more yang-oriented, like the bowel, stomach and bladder. Yin and yang organs work in pairs, like the stomach and the spleen. It is the smooth transition from one phase to another that is important, as well as the balance between the phases.

All of the organs are interrelated in their actions and reactions – the spleen is connected to the stomach and the pancreas, while the kidneys are seen as the 'mother' of the liver. The kidneys are also thought to balance the hormones, and to control teeth, bones and the hair of the head.

Still another concept vital to the proper balance in a body is 'qi' (pronounced 'chee'), which can be compared to a body's vital force. Qi is responsible for the physical, mental, emotional and spiritual processes of the body, and it moves along the twelve meridians that connect all parts of the body. Blood and body fluids are defined as a form of 'qi' – so is 'jing', which is stored in the kidneys and is similar in concept to a person's underlying constitution. In an emergency qi can be derived from jing. In Chinese medicine the emotions and the body are not separate, and a disorder in one affects the other. Again, a persons' good health is determined by maintaining a balanced, uninterrupted flow of qi. For one thing, it is qi which keeps the blood and body fluids circulating, so if the flow of qi is blocked, or in a state of imbalance, illness and pain may occur. The traditional Chinese model of disease believes that suppressed energy does not go away: it either becomes polluted, or the excessive build-up will give rise to symptoms. Qi also protects the body against wind, cold, damp and heat – that is, against environmental influence. For instance, qi will protect the body from getting too chilled from a cold wind, or from becoming stiff and aching from damp. A common cold, in Chinese medicine, is often referred to as an 'attack of cold wind' – this is a way of labelling how a condition manifests itself. Qi also protects against germs and viruses.

TREATMENT

The acupuncturist will ask you about your physical health as well as about your emotional and mental state, your work and your lifestyle in general. Your tongue will be looked at and your pulse taken in six places on each wrist (representing the twelve meridians) to determine the condition of your qi. The acupuncturist can also decide through these pulse points whether your mind as well as your body needs nourishment. After treatment, the acupuncturist may give you advice on diet, exercise and/or general lifestyle.

Treatment consists of gently inserting sterilised needles into acupuncture points which are chosen to increase or decrease either the yin or the yang forces. The usual places are on the forearms, hands, lower legs and feet. The points do not necessarily refer to the organs being treated, but to the channel along which these organs lie. There may be a pin-prick sensation, followed by a tingling, but there is usually no discomfort. The needles are solid but much finer than those used in orthodox medicine to give injections. They act like tuning forks, sending the right vibrations through the body.

A small cone of dried leaves of the herb moxa is then placed around the needle's head and lit, or a glowing moxa stick is held near the acupuncture point – this is to warm the needle, which in turn warms the qi in the channel being treated. The qi is thus activated to correct the imbalance that caused the illness. The needles are left in place an average of twenty minutes, but this can vary, depending on what disorder is being treated and on the training of the acupuncturist.

Treatment aims to get at the *root* of the problem, which may be an imbalance of yin yang, or of the five phases, or of the qi. During treatment, normal qi will be strengthened and disease-causing factors (such as phlegm, stagnant blood) will be dispelled. There are slightly different approaches to acupuncture, which is revealed in the way that diseases are categorised. A modern acupuncturist may work with a set of categories that is best for the patient, or use a combination of them.

According to acupuncturists, we all have a weakness in our bodies, whether it is genetic or is caused by diet or environment. In traditional Chinese medicine the four factors causing disease/imbalance in a person are diet, lifestyle, environment and unbalanced emotions. The psychological condition is the most important of the four factors in relation to cancer, because if this factor is damaged, the other three will not balance correctly. Qi and the blood and body fluids can all be undermined through an emotional disturbance, as well as by external conditions like cold, damp, heat and dryness, overwork, stress, bad diet or unhealthy lifestyle.

ACUPUNCTURE AND CANCER

Acupuncturists believe that most cancers involve emotional trauma. The liver is closely connected with the emotions, so an emotional trauma could cause an imbalance in this organ or vice versa. This could then create a 'domino' effect – the liver qi could become stagnated, which would then throw the yin energy out of balance, with subsequent blood stagnation, the production of phlegm in an attempt to dilute toxins and the generation of heat from the putrefaction. A cancer could then manifest itself as a growth within tissue or as a tumour deep within an organ. Dietary factors (which can cause phlegm and dampness) and an exhausting lifestyle (which weakens energy, leading to qi/blood stagnation) are also considered by acupuncturists to be contributing causes to cancer. To the Chinese, cancer is only a name, and what is important is the underlying imbalance which causes the symptoms.

Acupuncturists believe that if a body can acquire cancer, it can *de*-acquire it. A woman may find that her acupuncturist wants to take her off all other drugs before starting treatment, and she may want to get another opinion about this. For details on how to find an acupuncturist, see p.282.

CHINESE HERBS

Acupuncture works most strongly for a condition like cancer when it is combined with Chinese herbs. In China acupuncture and Chinese herbs are used alongside Western orthodox treatments to provide the most complete approach. Chinese herbs are all grown in China, and are very different from Western herbs. The way they work is even categorised differently, and they are very powerful, with specific actions. They are used to control malignant growths and to help the immune system, unlike Western herbs which are used only to strengthen the immune system. Clinical reports from China show some success with these herbs, but *how* they work is not known. It may be that they are in some way more toxic to the cancer cells than to healthy cells.

Acupuncture might be used first to improve the underlying strength of the patient, and then the more dynamic herbs would be used. There are many acupuncturists who also practice Chinese herbal medicine (you can find one in the Register of Chinese Herbal Medicine, listed on p.282). The herbs can move stagnation in the blood as well as in the liver qi and remove dampness and phlegm, while the acupuncture itself works more to improve the psyche. Stagnation in the liver qi can affect the uterus, ovaries and breast, and is also responsible for pre-menstrual symptoms, while blood stagnation can make periods clotty. 'Dampness' in the form of phlegm, mucus or fluid can build up to form masses, as well as cancerous tumours.

Treatment with Chinese herbs and acupuncture has helped women with various gynaecological problems, as well as those with CIN, early cervical cancer and breast cancer. The herbs can also help to reduce the side effects of chemotherapy and radiotherapy. Treatment works slowly and may take up to a year to complete its effects. Herbs are prescribed in a dried form; the patient boils them to make a tea which is then drunk once or twice a day. Sometimes powdered animal substances, such as shells, are also boiled up with the herbs.

Case Study – ACUPUNCTURE & CHINESE HERBAL MEDICINE

In 1982, at the age of forty-eight Jo Spence acknowledged that she had a breast lump which she'd ignored for a year. A needle biopsy drew nothing out and her mammogram was indecisive, so a sample of cells were taken for examination. The next thing Jo knew, she was admitted to hospital for a mastectomy, but she managed to convince her specialist to perform a lumpectomy only. The lump was found to be malignant. A biopsy of the lymph nodes in her neck and armpit was 'negative' as were a bone scan, liver scan and blood tests. No cancer spread could be seen.

Jo was still being advised to have a mastectomy, but instead she began looking hard at complementary therapies, visited the Bristol Centre and switched to a vegan diet. In 1983 Jo visited a naturopath but after nine months of treatment with natural herbs, a large lump rose in her left breast along with an 'orange peel' effect. The naturopath advised Jo to return to orthodox medicine, saying that she could do nothing more for her. Instead Jo went to an acupuncturist who used Chinese herbs. Although saying Jo was 'in bad shape', he agreed to take her on and she has stayed with him ever since.

Jo's remedies are changed as her symptoms change, but they usually consist of eight to twelve herbs, each with its own function. She boils the remedy up in a terracotta herb kettle to make a tea. According to her acupuncturist, the herbs act to break down tumour formation without the side effects that would accompany a treatment like chemotherapy. Sometimes herbs are given to liven up her system: at other times they are prescribed to slow her down. Although Jo admits that the Chinese herbal teas 'taste foul', she believes that they have strengthened her immune system, leaving her free of colds and flu; and, most important, the breast lump and orange-peel effect have disappeared.

Jo's breast cancer (and her lifelong battle against asthma) are viewed by her therapist as extensions of a chronic liver problem, and Jo plans to continue treatment to strengthen her lungs and liver. The treatment does take a lot out of her, though, and there are days when her energy levels are low. She now finds that she cannot tolerate orthodox medicine – even an aspirin seems to 'wipe out' her immune system. As a long-term patient, Jo gets a slight reduction in fees, but believes that every penny is worth it as she no longer feels that she is living on 'red alert'.

SCIENTIFIC ACUPUNCTURE AND PAIN RELIEF

'Scientific (or medical) acupuncture' is used by orthodox and complementary therapists alike to relieve pain – needles are applied to pressure points to stimulate the release of chemical endorphins from the brain. These naturally produced substances act like morphine to quell pain, interrupting the pain signals as they come up the spine. It is also believed that other chemicals involved in the transmission of nerve pulses are affected by acupuncture needles. While traditional acupuncture may be disputed in some camps, scientific acupuncture rarely is, and some NHS hospitals allow acupuncturists to treat for pain relief. The treatment is particularly useful for post-operative pain, where surgery has interfered with the channels through which energy passes.

HOMOEOPUNCTURE

As mentioned earlier, acupuncture and homoeopathy are the most alike of all the complementary therapies because they work on an 'energy' level. A combination of the two, 'homoeopuncture', is also practised by some therapists – it involves the dipping of acupuncture needles into homoeopathic remedies before inserting them into the skin.

Finding an acupuncturist

There are over 500 registered, non-medically qualified acupuncturists in Great Britain, and 600 doctors who use the technique. Fees vary and return visits would probably cost less than the initial consultation. The cost of herbs is extra. Part-time courses are available for those wishing to learn acupuncture, but a fully-qualified acupuncturist studies full-time for four years. If seeking treatments, be sure to find a qualified acupuncturist (see the list of addresses on p.282) as the art is in the diagnosis. However, a thorough knowledge of anatomy and of acupuncture points are also essential because care must be taken not to damage the blood vessels and the major organs.

14
Counselling and Relaxation Techniques

Complementary therapies are particularly good at helping a person on a mental, emotional and spiritual level, especially when an illness such as cancer is making life more difficult. Our physical body comes in for a lot of attention when we are ill, but often the person inside that body is ignored. Many patients suffer mentally much more than they suffer physically.

Cancer is not just a tumour growing inside us; it both affects how we feel physically and how we view ourselves, our relationships and the world in general; and it increases our stress and anxiety.

COUNSELLING

Counselling, which has already been mentioned (p.244), is an important part of the alternative approach to treating cancer. Studies have continually shown the importance of it: in one, up to 40 per cent of women were found to be suffering from depression, anxiety-neurosis and sexual problems after a mastectomy. Women with cancer may need someone professionally trained, with whom they can sort out their feelings. They may want to talk about deep-seated fears, related to dying and death, or the worry of leaving loved ones behind. They may want to explore sometimes unanswerable questions about *why* cancer has happened to them.

The issues that bubble to the surface with a disease like cancer sometimes never get discussed at any other time in a woman's life – it is as if the disease has acted as a catalyst to finding a solution to unanswered questions, forcing a person to gain a new perspective on her life and sort out her priorities. This is often too difficult to face up to alone, and it may not be enough just to talk to a friend or spouse. Some women may cope with their cancer well enough, but want help with other areas of stress in their lives, which may suddenly become too much for them to deal with.

At the Bristol Cancer Help Centre, counsellors experienced in the cancer field hold individual sessions. A counsellor's aim is three-fold: to help the patient release herself from emotional burdens; to discover the causes of stress, both past and present; and to encourage a more positive attitude.

Basically, a counsellor *listens* and, through hearing what you are saying, helps you to resolve or come to terms with a problem. You are encouraged to sort out your *own* thinking, and if a situation cannot be changed, it may be possible to change your reactions and attitude towards that situation. It may be that you need to face up to a part of yourself that you have been avoiding all your life, or that you need to vent your emotions in order to get rid of stress.

Sometimes it is just as necessary to allow ourselves to receive help as it is to help ourselves, and we mustn't be frightened, or feel unworthy to reach out to people who can help us. If you don't know of any counsellors in your area, the Bristol Centre may be able to give you contacts. (See also under 'Counselling' on p.284).

RELAXATION TECHNIQUES

Relaxing your body is all about recognising what tension feels like and 'letting go'. Without your realising it, cancer can stress your body into a permanent state of tension. The following relaxation exercise involves 'teaching' your body's muscle groups the difference between tension and relaxation, so that eventually your muscles learn to relax when you want them to.

All it takes is ten minutes, twice a day, although some relaxation experts advocate three half-hour sessions a day for cancer patients. See what you feel like doing, start off gently, and work up to the full-length exercise. Like anything else, the more you practise, the better you will become.

THE RELAXATION EXERCISE

First, find a comfortable chair in a quiet room, or lie on a bed. Take off your shoes and loosen any tight clothing. Choose some words or a phrase that will allow you to refocus your attention if it wanders during the exercise phrases such as 'I am still – still and becoming calm – becoming calm and still' are helpful. Then proceed as follows:

1. Keep your arms relaxed by your side with your palms down for a few minutes and feel yourself being quite still and sinking deeper into the chair or bed. Focus your eyes on a wall, or close them.
2. Take a deep breath, inhaling and exhaling on slow counts of five. Repeat this four times and repeat the words 'relax' silently to yourself each time you exhale. Imagine that all your cares and worries are leaving you on each exhalation.
3. Tense your face muscles by frowning as hard as you can, with eyes squeezed shut, for a slow count of five. Then relax your face muscles, noting the difference between tension and relaxation in such places as your eyebrows and the muscles around your eyes.
4. Next, tense your neck muscles by pushing your head firmly back against the chair or bed. All muscle tensing is done on the same count of five. Remember to continue breathing very regularly, repeating the word 'relax' on the exhale. When you relax, flop all the muscles completely.
5. Use the same technique on your shoulders – tense them by drawing them up as hard as possible, then relax.
6. Continue in the same way with your upper arms, forearms, hands, chest, stomach, thighs and calves, ending with your feet and toes. This whole procedure should take about nine minutes.
7. Once your body is completely physically relaxed, move on to relaxing your *mind*. Pick a soothing image, such as the countryside in spring, and fully explore this image for

about a minute, feeling all the colours, textures, smells and sounds.

You will know when you are completely relaxed because you will feel warm and heavy, with calm, regular breathing, no rapid eye movements, and a feeling of saliva in the mouth. To help you, relaxation tapes are available through several organisations, including the Bristol Centre and the ANAC (see the list of addresses on p.276).

BIO-FEEDBACK

Bio-feedback involves the use of a machine to tell you how relaxed or how stressed you are. It is a way of increasing your awareness of your own mental state by watching your body's responses. The various types of machine can measure such things as blood pressure, heart rate, temperature, brain-wave patterns and muscle tension; and the level of arousal of the nervous system can be revealed by measuring the electrical resistance of the skin.

The type of bio-feedback machine that measures skin resistance, for example, may consist of a small, black, electronic box, emitting a continuous tone or 'bleep', with a wire running from it. The wire is attached to two electrodes which are strapped to your palms: these measure changes in the body's surface moisture – for instance, when you are tense or anxious, you sweat more, and the machine picks up these changes and emits a higher tone. The tone falls away to a softer level when you are calm. Instead of or as well as a tone, on most models you can watch a needle on the box moving, from left to right, from 'relaxation' on the left to 'tension' on the right; and through relaxed concentration you can *will* yourself calmer so that the needle moves more towards the left. Other machines give feedback about your state of consciousness by emitting bleeps, so allowing you to keep your eyes closed. You can be trained to use the machine, and training usually starts with changing your reaction to stressful words. Training also instils an awareness of some of the skills and capabilities of the left and right brain hemisphere functions, and of the interactions between brain and body. Participants become more aware of their internal state. The machine can even be used to help you to control your own blood pressure.

Bio-feedback is a great way to learn to relax, and can be the precursor to deeper relaxation or meditation, during which healing at a deeper level may be taking place. If you wish to try a bio-feedback machine, a local woman's health group should know where you can rent one (see also p.283 for where to rent/buy a machine, and for training courses).

BREATHING

Deep, relaxed breathing (oxygenating) pumps more oxygen around the body and exchanges stale air for fresh, which helps the immune system, increases the sense of well-being, and calms both body and mind.

Oxygenating is a positive activity for health, even if doctors are uncertain if it affects cancer cells. You can do breathing exercises standing by an open window, sitting comfortably or lying down. You may want to do this after your relaxation exercise, when your body is completely relaxed. Follow the instructions below. (*NB: People with high blood pressure or a heart condition should not practise deep breathing.*)

1. Place your fingertips along the lower edge of your ribs, just above your waist at the front. The diaphragm (the muscular floor of the chest) attaches to this edge, and the lower part of the lungs lies just above the diaphragm. The upper part of each lung lies 2.5cm (1 inch) above each collarbone.
2. On a count of your choice, take a deep breath in through your nose with your mouth closed, feeling the abdomen and the lower ribs expand, then the middle ribs, followed by the upper chest. You might want to count along to your own heartbeat. Don't consciously raise the shoulders; let the breath lift the upper chest. The diaphragm is pulled downwards by this action and air is drawn into the lungs.
3. Hold the breath on the inhalation for the same count, which gives the air cells of the lungs longer to make an exchange

of fresh oxygen in return for carbon dioxide. This also helps to expand the lung capacity.

4. Exhale on the same count, feeling the diaphragm rising as air is expelled through the nostrils.

5. Hold again for the same count at the end of the breath, which improves the muscles surrounding the air cells by exercising them at the contraction end.

Repeat this breathing exercise ten times, working up to more repetitions if you like, and doing it several times a day. To keep the breath flowing more evenly and smoothly, imagine a feather a few inches from your nostrils which you don't want to disturb.

Details of other breathing exercises are available from the Bristol Centre, and are given in several books listed in the bibliography (see also p.283, 'Breathing Exercises').

15

Meditation, Visualisation and Spiritual Healing

Therapies that work on the mind may not be able to cure a cancer, but they can certainly add to a person's quality of life. However, for all we know, there may be even more to it than that. We are aware, for instance, that stress hormones (adrenalin and steroids) can remain in a person's bloodstream and disrupt the delicate chemical balance of the body's immune system. If these hormones remain in the bloodstream over a long period of time (indicating suppressed stress), they can interfere with the production of T-lymphocytes thus weakening the immune system.

MEDITATION

Meditation can be used to channel the power of the mind to help the body. Although it is usually associated with chanting hippies and orange-robed mystics from the East, it is simply a way of resting the mind and helping to 'centre' us in our daily lives by giving us a feeling of calm, poise and balance. Through meditation we can 'stand outside' ourselves and be our own observer, watching our body's and mind's reactions to daily events with more objectivity and detachment – and, ultimately, with more self-control. We can also detach ourselves from worry, fear and pain.

What happens first in meditation is that we concentrate on controlling our breathing, which allows outside stimuli to be shut out. Brain waves begin to slow down, switching from the beta waves of normal consciousness to the much slower waves of alpha consciousness, allowing the imaginative, intuitive side of our brain to dominate. This is the side of our brain usually beyond our conscious control. A sign that you have made this transition is a feeling of lightness in the body or of a light pressure band across the forehead or around the cheekbone area, sometimes accompanied by a tingling feeling. Blood pressure drops and breathing slows right down as the need for oxygen decreases. The individual is now in a trance-like state between sleeping and waking, where emotional blockages that may be holding up the healing process can be freed. Experienced yogis can control their blood pressure, heart rate and other bodily processes.

It is believed that the body is most receptive to healing suggestions in the meditative state, as it is freed from the distractions of everyday life. At the very least, meditation can bring you a new sense of inner peace and put you in touch with the wise inner being inside us all. And gradually, with practice, you will find that there is a flow-on effect from the meditation time into the bustle of your daily life.

Meditation can be started by counting breaths or repeating certain phrases, or 'mantras'. You need a quiet place to sit – sitting is better, as if you lie down you may be tempted to fall asleep! Find a place where you know that you won't be disturbed for at least twenty minutes. A darkened room is more relaxing and will help you to concentrate. Meditation requires dedication and discipline, and should be done daily at a fixed time. A good time to do it would be after relaxation and breathing exercises (see pp.245 – 248).

It is possible to teach yourself to meditate, but it is better to have a teacher. If you cannot find a teacher near you, a meditation tape may be helpful. A tape will also help you to 'time' your meditation. Some tapes take you through a complete meditation while others just provide background music to which you can meditate. You can obtain tapes from the organisations listed under 'Meditation' on p.288.

VISUALISATION

Visualisation is a powerful tool used by the self to heal the self – it gives power to the healing process through positive mental images, and is a way of holding a different image of reality in the mind – not a reality caught up with images of suffering, pain and death, but images of hope, healing and getting completely better. Developed by the American radiotherapist Carl Simonton, visualisation involves imagining your cancer cells to be any number of things that are weak and vulnerable, while your immune system is pictured to be all-powerful and de-vouring.

To visualise it's best to do relaxation first (see page 246), and then find an image that corresponds to your body healing itself, where your white blood cells are actively seeking out unwanted cells and getting rid of them.

For instance, the cancer cells could be visualised as minnows and your white blood cells as great white sharks gobbling them up; or your immune system could be visualised as a huge vacuum cleaner, sucking up all the dirty cancer cells. A more peaceful image is depicting your tumour as a block of ice, which the great warmth of your immune system is slowly melting, drop by drop. If your cancer is more widespread, you could picture your white blood cells glowing and moving slowly through your bloodstream sucking in any malignant cells. But the best images will come from your own imagination, what *you* are happiest working with. Whatever you choose, make sure that the last image in a visualisation session completely sweeps away the cancer – this way, you transcend the idea of getting 'a bit' better, to getting *all* better. You can also visualise while you're active: for instance, you could imagine plucking out another cancer cell while weeding the garden, or washing away another bad cell while doing the dishes. It's not just a technique to use while sitting down and concentrating hard; you can keep healing images at the back of your mind all the time and let them slip in and out of your thoughts.

Although this sounds like child's play, it has actually been shown to *work*: Carl and Stephanie Simonton's book *Getting Well Again* is full of case studies and testimonies about the way visualisation has helped towards a cancer remission or cure. The Simontons report that out of 159 cancer patients diagnosed as incurable who practised visualisation, sixty-three were alive two years later – and of those, fourteen had no evidence of cancer, twelve still had a tumour which was getting smaller and seventeen had a cancer that was stable. Although these results indicated only a short-term remission, visualisation is still considered by many doctors and therapists alike to be a valuable approach.

Visualisation is especially useful during chemotherapy and radiotherapy: some patients have experienced fewer side effects when they have visualised their treatments as doing them good. There seems to be truth in the maxim that if you think something is doing you good, it *will* do you good – such is the power of the mind. Although orthodox doctors will argue that all the evidence is most likely to be 'subjective', it is the patients themselves who say that visualisation is helpful – so perhaps it is not relevant that results are measured in a 'scientific' way. And it is just possible that one day scientists *will* be able to measure the effect that the mind has on the body.

Visualisation is a way of holding in the mind a different picture of reality, with the final image being a whole and healthy body – an image that must be held in our minds so that the body can aspire to it. At the Bristol Centre, two to three half-hour sessions of visualisation a day are recommended, but it might be easier to do a few minutes several times a day – this way, 'thinking' about cancer doesn't dominate so much of your time, which could be counterproductive and depressing for many women.

It would appear that 'imagining' yourself well *can* stimulate a healing response in the body, and however unknown the final outcome, it is still a positive weapon with which to arm yourself in the fight against cancer. After all, cancer is not just a 'physical' problem: it affects the whole person, so techniques like relaxation, breathing, meditation and visualisation should be used to try to strengthen the immune system and be used wholeheartedly.

Case Study – VISUALISATION

Katherina Collins decided to try visualisation after reading Carl Simonton's book. One of her fears was looking at the tumour in her left breast, so she decided to block out her left side completely and not even look at it or touch it. She visualised it as a block of ice that was slowly being melted by the sun (her immune system). Each drip of water represented another cancer cell gone. Katherina made herself really believe it; she knew that once the ice had melted she would be whole again. For the next three years she visited the Bristol Centre weekly, had Iscador injections (see p. 213) twice weekly and visualised like mad.

Then one day, while getting off a bus, she fell on her 'bad' side – this was the first physical contact she'd had with her left side in three years. Thinking that she might have damaged herself, she went to her GP and asked him to take a look. Gently he guided her hand to the affected breast – there was no tumour there. The growth had gone and the skin was whole again. Her 'positive' lymph nodes have not been retested, but Katherina instinctively knows that she is OK. Through visualisation she has developed a new communication with her body. She says, 'I felt compelled to follow my own instincts about my health and body. I never saw myself as a patient; I wanted to be in control.'

SPIRITUAL HEALING

Spiritual healing might be seen by some to smack of black magic, or to pre-suppose a belief in a Christian God – but neither supposition is true. Spiritual healing is actually the oldest therapy of all, the ancient tradition of the 'laying on of hands'. It is a gift that many of us possess to some extent, if only we knew how to tap it.

Research has shown that, when healing, healers have symmetrical alpha and theta brain-wave patterns not found in non-healers, and that they are capable of inducing the same symmetrical wave patterns in the brains of those being healed. Kirlian photography, which has captured the energy fields surrounding plants and animals, has also managed to photograph the increased energy that comes from a healer's hands.

Healers see themselves as channels through which healing energy can flow: some healers believe that the energy comes from God; others believe it comes from energy fields present in the universe. Healers apparently have something in their energy fields which is able to interact with the energy fields of their patients and in some way reinvigorate these fields – although how this happens is not known. It may be due to some biological factor which has yet to be discovered.

Some healers actually touch the afflicted part, while others just pass their hands over the whole body from a distance of a few inches (called 'stroking'), lingering over those parts where there appears to be less warmth. Some healers work on your 'aura' (the energy field that surrounds your body and which some people can *see*), while others concentrate on specific 'chakras' (energy centres) of the body. 'Charismatic healing' is practised by the Charismatic Christians (from the teachings of St Luke) who believe that they can also help to release spiritual powers in a person. 'Distant healing' involves spiritual healers sending healing thoughts to a person who is somewhere else – even on the other side of the world! Some healers concentrate on being the 'middleman' between the patient and God. Often a person can feel a warm, tingling sensation while receiving healing; at the very least she feels relaxed, peaceful and serene after healing. Be sure to find a healer whom you can trust, and be wary of any who charge you large sums of money: most healers give healing free, or ask for a small donation. Be wary also of any healer who promises a cure.

Receiving healing is reputed to increase and accelerate our own natural healing ability, increase physical energy, help with pain and bring greater clarity of mind, calmness and peace. Healers believe that healing can take place without the patient believing in it; but some cancer patients think that believing has helped their cancer to diminish. Some healers have been shown to affect animals and plants and even laboratory-grown cells, but how this is done is not clear.

Healers are one of the few groups allowed into NHS hospitals: in fact, the Confederation of Healing Organisations recently launched a five-year project in NHS hospitals throughout the country to evaluate how spiritual healing affects certain illnesses, including cataracts, rheumatoid arthritis and cancer in young children – all diseases which orthodox doctors find hard to cure. The healers will also be helping to lessen pain during this project, and the overall results will be evaluated by independent medical scientists. To find a spiritual healer, look under 'Spiritual Healing' on p.191.

Case Study – SPIRITUAL HEALING
June Rogers is a spiritual healer who had a bladder tumour: during her brief bout with cancer she both received spiritual healing and gave

it out to others. Her mother and grandmother were clairvoyants and spiritual healers and June believes that she has inherited their gifts. Her healing is based on a belief in God: working through the 'spirit' of God while healing others means that she doesn't have to draw on her own energies. In fact she always ends up refreshed after a session, because the passage of the healing spirit through her 'always leaves a little bit behind'.

Her healing action involves mentally splitting the healing intention into different-coloured rays, depending on the type of condition being treated: red, blue, pink, gold and green are her colours, and each feels different to give or to receive — some feeling warm, hot or even cold. Her healing 'guides' decide which colour will be used when healing someone — June feels herself to be only the 'instrument' through which healing power from God flows. June was also able to give herself healing, and received healing regularly from other healers, in the three-month time limit she gave herself to rid her body of the bladder tumour. And June's efforts succeeded (see the case study on p.179).

16
Summing Up

You may now have an understanding of what the orthodox treatments are for women's cancers and how they work: surgery, radiotherapy, chemotherapy, hormone therapy, some forms of immunotherapy and counselling. You may also have an appreciation of the complementary approach, which includes physical therapies (diet, vitamins and minerals, enzymes, supplements, immunotherapy, detoxification, relaxation and breathing exercises); mental therapies (counselling, meditation, visualisation); spiritual therapy (spiritual healing); and those holistic therapies that address every level of a woman with a female cancer (herbalism, homoeopathy and acupuncture). When any combination of alternative therapies is taken alongside orthodox treatments, it is called the 'complementary' approach.

Cancer, with its many variations, is a great challenge to any therapy – and it may be through the combination of both the orthodox and complementary methods that the greatest cancer cures will be achieved. Both approaches are part of a greater whole, that whole being the sum of viable treatments that will help a woman with one of the female cancers.

THE CANCER DIAGNOSIS

If you have been given a cancer diagnosis, don't panic. Try to keep calm: it is your body, and you are still in control. As Penny Brohn says, it is possible for cancer to be in a body, but for the body to be in control of it. Before rushing off to the nearest specialist to present him/her with your problem, first examine your own feelings and think through how *you* would like to see it resolved. Then go out and collect the information you can from doctors, specialists, cancer organisations, complementary therapies and their organisations, and from other cancer patients. Check your facts, and get second or third opinions where necessary – or, if you are feeling overwhelmed, get someone to help you do this. Listen to other people's advice, but feel free to reject it. Visit a specialist in your kind of cancer and tape the interview if possible.

Bring with you a long list of questions that you have had ample time to prepare. Bring a friend or your spouse with you, to give you the courage to ask these questions, or to jog your memory where necessary.

If your condition isn't immediately life-threatening, explore the possibilities of complementary therapies that appeal to you. Very few cancers spread like wildfire, so you should have time in which to make enquiries. If you need surgery, get yourself referred to the best surgeon for your kind of cancer. Above all, *think positive*. This might be difficult to do at the beginning. As one ovarian cancer patient put it, 'At first, thinking and acting positive was an "act" for me, but as time went on and treatments were successful, my confidence was boosted and the positive outlook became a part of my personality.'

According to one doctor, only you know what you feel, what is important to you and what price you would be prepared to pay for possible recovery. You will be making decisions about your treatment based on expert advice combined with your own unique knowledge of yourself.

Become *involved* with your fight for recovery by looking at ways in which you can change your diet to a more healthy one, at ways to relieve stress and increase your feelings of self-control and well-being. Let your family help you by telling them what you need, both physically and emotionally. Contact your local cancer self-help group for support. In the early days you may feel that you have become obsessed with your illness, its treatment and yourself, but this is only natural – as time passes, you will find that all of this has 'taken a back seat' to the rest of your life. What you *don't* want to do is to end up with a lifestyle that is aimed solely at fighting cancer, which leaves with you little else in the way of living.

In the end cancer must be put in perspective: four-fifths of all deaths in general are due to causes other than cancer. Life and death themselves must be put in perspective: it is the eternal balancing act that each and every one of us struggles with. As Audre Lorde, author of *The Cancer Journals* remarks, it's about 'looking death in the face and not shrinking from it, but never embracing it too easily'. Cancer patients may suffer physically and mentally with their illness, but they often learn things and gain a wider perspective than was possible before they were ill. As Vicky Clement-Jones, a doctor and ovarian cancer sufferer said, 'I learnt something about myself during my illness. I learnt about how precious life was and how I wanted to live my life. I learnt about my relationships with my friends and family and how important they were to me, and how the illness had brought us closer together. I was surprised to find that life could be enriched by such traumatic illness. Somehow the experience of my personal struggle with the illness had sharpened my focus on life. I reorganised my priorities and had a new zest for life, living each day as it came.'

THE PROS AND CONS OF ORTHODOX AND COMPLEMENTARY TREATMENTS

It is sometimes too easy to knock the complementary therapies for lack of scientific 'proof' – though that proof may yet be forthcoming. Orthodox methods get knocked as well, for the unsubtlety of their cut/burn/poison approach. But it is easy to forget how much we owe orthodox medicine and its scientific procedures: for instance, if it weren't for clinical trials, we would never have known that lumpectomy is as good as a radical mastectomy for some breast cancers. Scientific evaluation, where possible, should always be encouraged, because it has brought in its wake great medical advances.

Orthodox medicine is now looking at the emotional, mental and spiritual resources of cancer patients to see if they can be harnessed in some way to promote a cure. Says Professor Baum, 'If it exists, then we will find a way to measure it.' If faith can help to make a person whole, perhaps one day science will understand the mechanism.

Although many of the complementary therapies seem much more effective as 'preventatives' than as 'cures' at the present time, evidence linking such things as diet to cancer is mounting constantly, and the tentative links between personality, stress and cancer, may yet be strengthened by future research. The way to *measure* the success rates of various complementary therapies may be just around the corner, and cancer patients will be forgiven for not wanting to wait years for 'absolute' proof when their health or their life is on the line.

FUTURE BRIDGES BETWEEN ORTHODOX AND COMPLEMENTARY TREATMENTS

One of the future bridges between orthodox and complementary treatments may be 'electromagnetic medicine', in which molecular scanners perceive a pre-cancerous state through energy imbalances before there are even symptoms, and other electromagnetic machines will pulse energy back into the parts of the body where it is needed. This is actually an extension of physics medicine, which addresses the body on a molecular level. Along with nutritional guidelines, this could be the treatment of tomorrow, where drugs are rarely used – and when they are, their side effects are minimised by the use of other 'holistic' therapies. Another bridge between the camps could be the further development of immunotherapy, with the immune system stimulated to complete the battle against cancer all by itself.

At the moment, however, some orthodox hospitals are making available to cancer patients therapies that have previously been available only from complementary medical centres or therapists. At the Hammersmith Hospital in London, for example, a liaison was set up with the Bristol Cancer Help Centre in mid-1989. Patients and their relatives and friends at the Hammersmith Cancer Centre are offered an opportunity to meet weekly with a support group, as well as counselling and lessons on relaxation and visualisation techniques. For information on other therapies such as dietary changes, acupuncture, homoeopathy and spiritual healing, patients and their relatives are asked to contact the Bristol Cancer Help Centre directly.

Check what is available in the way of cancer support activities at your nearest big hospital – if there isn't much on offer, perhaps you could help to instigate or organise the creation of more self-help facilities there.

CURRENT NEEDS OF FEMALE CANCER PATIENTS

All of this will be good news for women with a 'female' cancer, and for their families and friends, but what these women need even more, and what they need *now*, is a medical system that encourages early diagnosis and preventative treatment, and a health system in which they can make more informed choices about what is most suitable for them.

Five-year survival rates need redefining, to embrace a much wider definition of success that includes, for example, quality of life. Therapists on *both* sides of the fence must learn to tell women the whole truth about their respective treatments, without oversized egos and vested interests getting in the way. As one medically-trained therapist put it, 'The problem is that there are no experts; only people who *think* they are experts.'

Both orthodox and complementary therapies should be available to *all* women: the choice should not be dictated by where a woman lives or by how much she can afford. This will mean a coming together of orthodox and complementary medicine in new ways, with the sole aim of returning a person to full health. This is something that all healthy women should be working towards, and to which all 'unwell' women should be entitled: the freedom to choose the best set of treatments under the best, unbiased guidance from both sides for her particular cancer.

Glossary of Terms

Abnormal smear A smear result showing an abnormality, such as inflammatory changes, CIN or an infection of the cervix.

Adenocarcinoma A cancer starting in glandular tissue.

Adjuvant treatment A secondary treatment which usually follows surgery and involves chemotherapy or radiotherapy. It is given if your cancer has an inclination to relapse, even if at the time it is given there are no symptoms.

Aflatoxin One of a number of toxic carcinogenic substances resembling mould which may contaminate badly stored foods (such as peanuts).

Alteratives Those herbs which cleanse and normalise when used on tumours.

Aminoglutethimide A drug used in the treatment of hormone-receptive breast cancers, which inhibits oestrogen formation by suppressing the action of the adrenal glands.

Anaerobic Living in the absence of free oxygen.

Analgesic Medicine to control pain.

Anti-coagulant An agent that prevents the clotting of blood.

Antigen Any substance that the body regards as foreign or potentially dangerous, and against which it produces an antibody.

Anti-neoplastics Herbs blocking new growth when used on a tumour.

Anti-oxidant Any substance which protects against decomposition. It includes certain enzymes and vitamins which can prompt cancer cells to repair themselves, and can help produce more antibodies.

Areola The dark area surrounding the nipple.

Atrophy The wasting away of a normally developed organ or tissue as a result of the degeneration of cells, such as the shrinking of the ovaries at the menopause.

Attenuation Reduction of the virulence of a bacterium or virus by chemical treatment, heating, drying, by growing under adverse conditions or by passing through another organism. This is done for many immunisations.

Auto-immune disease Inflammation and destruction of tissues by the body's own antibodies.

Axilla Armpit.

Bacillus Aerobic, rod-shaped bacterium; any disease-causing bacterium.

Barium enema Special X-ray of the bowel.

Barrier methods of contraception Those which stop sperm from getting on to the cervix, that is, the cap or diaphragm and the condom.

Benign Used to describe a tumour which may interfere with body functions and require removal, but which does not invade neighbouring tissue.

Bilateral salpingo-oophorectomy Removal of both ovaries.

Bi-manual pelvic examination An examination in which the doctor uses two hands to examine the woman's lower abdomen and internal organs via the vagina and rectum.

Bio-flavinoids Natural substance found in vitamin C which aids absorption.

Biopsy Diagnosis by cutting out a piece of suspect tissue and examining it under a microscope.

Blood count The number of cells in a sample of blood.

B-lymphocyte A type of white blood cell originating from the bone marrow which produces antibodies.

Body scan *See* Computer-assisted tomography scan.

Bone scan A test to see if cancer has spread to the bones.

Breasts Glands formed mainly from fatty tissue, containing a system of ducts which carry milk to the nipple for feeding a baby.

Breast reconstruction Making a new breast after a mastectomy. A combination of muscle and skin from another part of the body and a silicone implant are used.

Breast self-examination (BSE) A procedure for examining the breasts for any sign of abnormality that could be the start of a cancer. Should be performed every month by all women.

Caesium A silver-white, soft, alkaline metal used in compounds or alloys of photo-electric cells.

Caesium 137 An artificial radioactive isotape of the metallic element caesium; the radiation it gives off is used in radiotherapy.

Cancer Not a single disease with a single cause and single type of treatment, but more than 200 different kinds of disease, each with its own name and treatment.

Carboplatin The newest platinum-derived compound used in chemotherapy to treat ovarian cancer. It has the same action as cisplatin, but causes less nausea. Also known as JM8.

Carcinogen A chemical that will cause cancer in animals.

Carcinoma A cancer that develops from cells called epithelial cells, present in the skin, lungs, glands and gastro-intestinal and urinary tracts. It is the commonest type of cancer.

Carcinoma in situ Cancer cells which are localised, confined to the surface tissue and not invasive. Included in CIN 3.

Case-control study Comparison of a group of people who have a disease with another group free from that disease. In the more precise 'matched pair' study, every individual with the disease is paired with a control matched on the basis of, for example, age, sex or occupation, in order to place greater emphasis on a factor for which the pairs have not been matched.

CAT Scan *See* Computer-assisted tomography scan.

Catheter Instrument used for the passage of fluids, usually from the bladder.

Cauterisation A treatment using an electric probe to burn and destroy abnormal cells in the cervix.

Cell The smallest unit of the body capable of independent life.

Cervical canal Passage in the cervix that connects the main part of the uterus with the upper vagina.

Cervical dysplasia *See* Dysplasia.

Cervical erosion An abnormal area of surface tissue that may develop at the neck of the womb as a result of tissue damage caused at childbirth or by attempts at abortion.

Cervical intra-epithelial neoplasia Abnormal cells on the surface of the cervix, which are either CIN 1 (mild), CIN 2 (moderate) or CIN 3 (severe).

Cervicography A special camera with a light source (or 'cervicography') which can illuminate and photograph the cervix.

Cervix The lower, narrow end of the uterus that projects into the upper vagina.

Chelating agent A chemical compound that forms complexes by binding metal ions. It often forms the active centre of an enzyme.

Chemotherapy The use of cytotoxic (cancer-destroying) drugs. These drugs combine with and then damage the genetic material of cells, so that they can't divide properly.

Chromosome One of the threadlike structures in a cell nucleus that carry inheritance information in the form of genes.

CIN *See* Cervical intra-epithelial neoplasia.

Cisplatin A platinum-derived compound used in chemotherapy to treat ovarian cancer.

Co-carcinogen A chemical that is not in itself cancer-causing, but which can somehow provoke another chemical to cause cancer.

Cold coagulation A treatment involving a heated probe being put on to the surface of the cervix to burn abnormal cells.

Colposcopy An examination of the cervix through a binocular microscope (or 'colposcope'), which magnifies the cervix and makes it easy to see where the abnormal cells are.

Columnar cells Column-shaped cells which produce mucus. These cells mainly line the canal leading from the vagina into the uterus.

Complementary Used to describe all the alternative forms of medicine, such as homoeopathy, herbalism and acupuncture, with an emphasis on co-operation with orthodox medicine.

Computer-assisted tomography (CAT) scan A computer-produced picture which resembles 'slices' through different parts of the body. An electronic X-ray detector is used instead of the usual film, and the X-ray source rotates around the patient. All the information is then processed by computer, and a three-dimensional picture can be made. Also known simply as a body scan.

Cone biopsy Removal of a cone-shaped wedge of abnormal tissue from the cervix for microscopic analysis. The piece removed is only 1½ cm (about ½ inch) deep and the procedure is done under general anaesthetic.

Consultant Senior hospital doctor.

Cryosurgery The use of a special probe to freeze and destroy abnormal tissue on the surface of the cervix without harming the normal surrounding tissues. Also known as cryotherapy.

Cyst An abnormal sac or closed cavity filled with liquid or semi-solid matter. If a breast, it is a small sac of fluid which originates from the milk-producing glands.

Cytotoxic Used to describe a drug that damages or destroys cells and is employed in treating various types of cancer. It kills cancer by inhibiting cell division, but can also affect normal cells, particularly in the bone marrow, skin and stomach lining. The dosage must be carefully controlled.

Deoxyribonucleic acid (DNA) The genetic material of nearly all living organisms which controls heredity and is located in the nucleus of every cell.

Diagnosis The process of determining the nature of a disorder by considering the patient's symptoms, medical background and the results of any tests.

Diathermy The removal of abnormal cells in the cervix by passing a tiny electric current through the affected area.

Dilatation and curretage A scraping of cells from the uterus for microscopic examination. Under a general anaesthetic the cervix is expanded (dilatation) just enough to permit the insertion of a small instrument that removes material from the uterine lining (curettage).

DNA *See* Deoxyribonucleic acid.

Duct A tubelike structure or channel which carries glandular secretions.

Dyskaryosis Abnormalities seen in the cells taken in a cervical smear. It is included in the term 'CIN'.

Dyspareunia Painful sex.

Dysplasia The presence of abnormal cells in the surface layer of the cervix. Cervical dysplasia can be classified as 'mild', 'moderate' or 'severe'. It is included in the term 'CIN', but it also gives information about the cell abnormalities that can only be seen in a biopsy.

Electrolyte The concentration of ions (atoms that conduct electricity) in the bloodstream. They can be lost from the body by vomiting or diarrhoea.

Empirical Results based on observation, not theory.

Emulsified When fine droplets of one liquid (such as oil) are dispersed in another liquid (such as water), the first liquid is described as 'emulsified'.

Endocrine glands (ductless glands) Glands manufacturing hormones and secreting them into the bloodstream, not through a duct. Examples are pituitory, thyroid, adrenals, ovary, placenta.

Endocrine therapy The use of hormones to treat disease. Known also as hormone therapy.

Endometrium The lining of the uterus.

Endorphins Chemical compounds that occur naturally in the brain and have pain-relieving properties similar to those of opiate drugs (such as morphine).

Enzymes Biochemical compounds which oversee the organisation and arrangement of living matter without changing themselves. They are catalysts, and exert their own electrical fields.

Epithelial Surface-lining.

Examination under anaesthetic (EUA) Procedure carried out if cervical cancer is suspected when the abnormal cells are out of vision.

The cervix and other female organs are examined under a general anaesthetic.

Excision biopsy Removing a whole breast lump under general anaesthetic for examination.

External radiotherapy When used in connection with breast cancer, this involves the planting of wires made from irridium into the affected breast under a local or a general anaesthetic to give an extra dose of radiation to the area around the tumour.

Fallopian tubes The pair of tubes, one each side of the top of the uterus, which conduct the egg from the ovary to the uterus.

False negative The name given to any cancer that occurs within twelve months of a negative screening test. Some cancers may have been missed, and others may have started in between screenings and then grown quickly.

False positive This is when screening or testing reveals what appears to be a cancerous lump or growth, but surgery reveals it to be benign.

Fibroadenoma Small, fibrous lump of glandular tissue.

Fibroblast A cell in connective tissue that is responsible for the production of the first stage of collagen and elastic fibres.

Fibrotic Unwholesome growth of fibrous tissue.

Free radicals Supercharged molecules resulting from normal life processes which are unstable due to the loss of an electron and which disrupt other cells in their attempt to regain an electron.

Frozen section The taking of a small slice of breast lump during surgery, which is then rushed to a laboratory for analysis. If malignant cells are found, the operation becomes a mastectomy, combining two operations in one.

Gamma globulin Any one of a class of proteins present in the blood plasma, identified by their characteristic rate of movement in an electric field. Almost all gamma globulins are immuno-globulins.

Gamma radiation Electromagnetic radiation of wavelengths shorter than X-rays, given off by certain radioactive substances. It has greater penetration than X-rays.

Gene A unit of inheritance, which carries the chemical blue print for correct cell reproduction.

Germ-cell tumour A tumour arising from any of the embryonic cells that have the potential to develop into sperm or eggs.

Grade The measure of how aggressive a cancer is. It can be discovered by looking at a sample of the cancer cells under a microscope.

Heart fibrillation A rapid and chaotic beating of the many individual muscle fibres of the heart, making it unable to maintain properly timed contractions. The affected part of the heart then ceases to pump blood.

Herpes virus One of a group of DNA-containing viruses causing latent infection in men and animals, including the infections herpes and chicken pox. The group also includes the Epstein-Barr virus.

Holism A belief that the mind, body and spirit cannot be seen as separate entities.

Hormone A chemical messenger that circulates in the blood to control the growth and metabolism of tissue.

Hormone Replacement Therapy (HRT) A combination of the hormones oestrogen and progesterone given to women with missing or inactivated ovaries, or to women after the menopause, to stop such menopausal symptoms as osteoporosis and heart disease.

Hormone therapy The use of hormone drugs which inhibit the growth of women's cancers, like those of the uterus and breast, that are sensitive to messages from hormones.

Hyperplasia The increased production and growth of normal cells in tissue or an organ, such as the breasts during pregnancy. The affected part becomes larger, but retains its normal form.

Hysterectomy The surgical removal of the uterus; sometimes the cervix, Fallopian tubes and ovaries are removed as well.

Immuno-globulin One of a group of structurally related proteins that act as antibodies.

Immunology The study of immunity and all the phenomena connected with the defence mechanisms of the body.

Immunotherapy The prevention or treatment of disease using agents that may modify the immune response. It is largely an experimental approach, studied mostly in connection with cancer.

Inflammatory changes Cell damage caused by bacteria, viruses, IUD strings, etc., but which are *not* CIN.

In situ Only in one place. Used to describe the earliest stage of a cancer, when it stays where it has started.

Interferon A substance that is produced by cells infected by a virus, which has the ability to inhibit viral growth. Interferons only work in the species that product them. Attempts are being made now to produce human interferon in large amounts in bacterial host cells.

Interleukin 2 A hormone that directs a type of white blood cell called a T-lymphocyte.

Interleukin 3 A substance unrelated to Interleukin 2, which directs a blood cell called a 'polymorph' that eats cancer cells.

Internal radiation Treatment which consists of small radioactive packets resembling tampons being placed in the vagina for short periods of time to combat cervical cancer.

Intravenous pyelogram (IVP) or intravenous urogram (IVU) A test used to see if a tumour is interfering with the urinary system. An iodine compound is injected into a vein and is studied by X-ray as it passes through the kidneys, down the ureters and into the bladder.

Invasive cancer Cancerous cells that are growing beyond the surface layer of the organ and into other tissue.

Labia majora The larger, outer pair of lip-shaped skin folds that enclose the vulva.

Labia minora The smaller, inner pair of fleshy 'lips' that enclose the vulva.

Langerhams' cells Cells which fight infection and are that part of the immune system which specifically recognises viral infections and creates an immune response to them.

Laparoscopy A small operation which allows doctors to look through a mini-telescope (or 'Laparoscope') and take a small tissue sample for examination.

Laparotomy An operation to remove ovarian cancer. A 'second look' laparotomy is when a second operation is done at some point after the first in order to check that all the cancer is gone.

Laser therapy The use of a laser to vaporise abnormal cervical cells by an intense beam of laser light.

Leukocyte (or leucocyte) A white blood cell found in the lymph nodes, spleen, thymus gland, gut wall and bone marrow.

Liver ultrasound scan A test using ultrasound to see if cancer has spread to the liver.

Lobule A small, separate subdivision of breast tissue.

Localised All in one place.

Local recurrence A tumour that reappears at the site of the original tumour.

Lumpectomy In cases of breast cancer, the removal of the affected part of the breast with some armpit lymph nodes for testing.

Lymph A colourless fluid contained in blood plasma that passes through capillary walls, bathing tissue cells, nourishing them and removing waste products. Also found in the lymphatic vessels.

Lymphatic system Circulatory network of vessels throughout the body which carry lymph. The system also consists of the lymph nodes, spleen and thymus gland, which produces and stores infection-fighting cells.

Lymphatic vessels Vein-like structures that carry lymph around the body.

Lymph nodes Small glands the size of a bean which connect to the lymphatic system through which the lymph flows. They act as a filtering system and contribute to the body's defences against injury and disease. If a stray cancer cell gets trapped in a lymph node, the lymphatic system is blocked and the system transmits the malignancy.

Lymphocyte A type of white blood cell whose function is to identify and destroy invaders.

Lymphoedema An accumulation of lymph in the tissues.

Lymphogram or lymphangiogram An X-ray procedure to see if any lymph nodes are affected by disease.

Magnetic resonance scanning Painless, new, sophisticated technique which measures the water content of tissues. Cancer growths have a different water content from healthy tissue and so give off different signals.

Malignant Used to describe a tumour that invades or destroys surrounding normal tissue.

Mammography A special X-ray process that can detect abnormalities in the breast and differentiate between malignant and benign tumours.

Mastectomy An operation to remove part or all of a breast in which there is cancer. A partial mastectomy takes only the tumour and a wedge of normal tissue around it. A simple mastectomy takes the affected breast and the armpit glands. A modified radical mastectomy takes the breast, underarm lymph nodes and the lining over the chest muscles. A radical mastectomy takes the breast, armpit glands, chest muscles and some fat and skin.

Mega-vitamins High doses of vitamins given for therapeutic reasons.

Menopause The time in a woman's life when the ovaries stop producing an egg every four weeks and menstruation stops. It occurs any time from the mid-thirties to the late fifties.

Metaplasia During adolescence, pregnancy and when on the contraceptive pill, columnar cells on the surface of the cervix are replaced by sqyamous cells. This process, which takes place in the transformation zone, is normal cell growth.

Metastasis The process during which cancer cells break away from the tumour and spread through the bloodstream or lymphatic system to distant parts of the body, where they form new cancers.

Micro sievert Measure of radiation dose.

Mild dysplasia The condition in which abnormal cells are found only in the bottom third or less of the surface layer of the cervix. Also known as CIN 1.

Moderate dysplasia The condition in which abnormal cells are found in the bottom third to two-thirds of the surface layer of the cervix. Also known as CIN 2.

Monoclonal antibody An antibody produced artificially in a laboratory by fusing lymphocytes from mouse spleen with mouse cancer cells.

Morbidity Symptoms or effects of a disease or its treatments.

Multifactorial Used to describe conditions believed to have resulted from the interaction of genetic and environmental factors.

Multifocal In many different places.

Mutation Change in genetic structure.

Needle aspiration Drawing off fluid from a breast lump for microscopic examination.

Needle biopsy Removing solid cells from a breast lump for microscopic examination.

Neoplasm A new and abnormal growth; any benign or malignant tumour.

Neuro-endocrine system The system of dual control of certain activities of the body by means both of nerves and circulating hormones. The functioning of the autonomic nervous system is particularly closely linked to that of the pituitary and the adrenal glands.

Nitrate A salt of nitric acid, which is used as an agricultural fertiliser.

Nitrite A salt of nitrous acid, which is used as an agricultural fertiliser.

Non-invasive cells Cancerous cells that have not yet begun to grow into surrounding tissue.

Nuclear magnetic resonance (NMR) A technique used in the diagnosis of brain abnormalities, vascular disease and cancer. Based on the absorption of specific radio frequencies by atomic nuclei, it enables the imaging of parts of the body in any plane.

Nulliparity The state of not giving/never having given birth to a child.

Occult tumour A hidden or concealed tumour.

Oestrogen A hormone produced naturally in a woman's body mainly by the ovaries, promoting the growth and function of the female sex organs and female secondary sex characteristics.

Oncogene A gene in viruses and in the cells of mammals that can cause cancer. It probably produces proteins regulating cell division that, under certain circumstances, becomes uncontrolled.

Oncologist A tumour specialist.

Oncology The study and practice of treating tumours.

Os The entrance to the canal that passes through the cervix from vagina to uterus. It is the pathway for sperm, blood and babies.

Osteoporosis The loss of bony tissue, resulting in bones that are brittle and liable to fracture. It is common in the elderly and in women following the menopause.

Ovaries Two egg-producing glands the size of olives, located on each side of the uterus.

Ozone A form of oxygen with three oxygen atoms per molecule; it is a very powerful oxidising agent formed when oxygen or air is subjected to electric discharge. Ozone is found in the atmosphere at very high altitudes and is responsible for destroying a large proportion of the sun's ultraviolet radiation.

Palliative treatment Treatment aimed to kill pain rather than to cure.

Palpable Capable of being felt.

Parametrium The layer of connective tissue surrounding the womb.

Pathology The branch of medicine concerned with the study of disease.

Pelvic area The area of the body lying within the pelvic bone. Organs in this area include the uterus, vagina, ovaries, Fallopian tubes, bladder and rectum.

Peptide A molecule consisting of two or more amino acids.

Peritoneoscopy A procedure used to see if there is any cancer left after surgery, using a tiny microscope. It is carried out under local anaesthetic.

Peritoneum The covering membrane of the abdominal cavity.

Pharmacology The science of drugs.

Photochemical therapy The combination of light with certain substances which can select and destroy tumour cells while leaving normal cells relatively unharmed. Also called light therapy.

Physiology The science of the functioning of living organisms and of their component parts.

Pituitary gland The endocrine gland at the base of the brain which controls many of the other endocrine glands.

Platelets Cells in the blood which help it to clot.

Positive smear A term without a universally agreed definition, but it usually means the same as CIN.

Pre-cancerous cells Abnormally shaped cells that are one stage away from being cancer.

Pre-malignant Used to describe an abnormal area in the body that may or may not develop into a cancer.

Primary A cancer present at the site in which it developed.

Progesterone A hormone produced naturally in a woman's body by the adrenal gland, the ovaries and the placenta; it is responsible for preparing the womb lining for pregnancy.

Progestogen One of a group of naturally occurring or synthetic steriod hormones, including progesterone, that maintains the normal course of pregnancy.

Prognosis An assessment of the future course and outcome of a patient's disease, based on knowledge of the course of the disease in other patients, together with the general health, age and sex of the patient. It is generalised from the progress of many patients and cannot accurately predict the outcome for an individual.

Prolactin A pituitary hormone that stimulates milk production. It can be produced in excess as a result of stress when women face breast surgery.

Prophylactic Treatment designed to prevent a disease.

Prophylactic oophorectomy The surgical removal of the ovaries as a preventative measure.

Prostaglandins A group of essential fatty acids which affect the nervous system, circulation, female reproductive organs and metabolism.

Prosthesis An artificial breast that can be worn in a bra after a mastectomy.

Proteolytic A digestive enzyme that causes the breakdown of protein.

Punch biopsy Cutting out a very small piece of tissue to be tested, which is done during a colposcopy.

Radiation therapy or radiotherapy The treatment of cancer by X-rays which destroy the cancer cells near the surface of the body. A beam of radiation is focused on the cancer and kills it without affecting normal tissue. Cobalt, radium and caesium are some of the sources used. By itself radiotherapy can cure some breast, some cervix and some uterine cancers.

Radioactive implants The use of radioactivity in a limited area, such as on the breast in the form of a grid of irridium wires, or in the uterus with tubes resembling tampons filled with a radioactive substance. It gives a large dose to the tumour, and as small a dose as possible to the surrounding tissue. (*See* also Internal radiotherapy.)

Radio-isotope scanning The measurement of the way in which different parts of the body absorb different chemicals when made radioactive. The radioactive chemicals, or isotopes, cause an emission which can reveal an abnormality in the area in question.

Randomised controlled trial Trial (of, say, a new cancer treatment) in which people are allocated to their respective groups by means of random numbers. The 'control' group has no active treatment.

Recurrence A cancer that occurs again at a later date in the same place as the original, treated cancer.

Registrar Middle-ranking hospital doctor.

Relapse The regrowth of a cancer after it has been removed or has responded to treatment.

Remission Shrinkage of a tumour, partially or wholly, but which doesn't necessarily indicate a cure.

Replication The process by which DNA makes copies of itself when a cell divides.

Ribonucleic acid (RNA) A nucleic acid occurring in the nucleus and cytoplasm of cells that is concerned with the synthesis of proteins. In some viruses, RNA is the genetic material.

Schiller test The application of iodine to the cervix; the normal areas are darkened by the iodine, and the abnormal parts are not.

Secondary A cancer that has developed in an area different from where it first started.

Segmentectomy Another term for partial mastectomy, which removes a breast tumour and a wedge of normal tissue around it.

Severe dysplasia (CIN 3) The condition in which abnormal cells cover at least two-thirds but not the entire surface layer of the cervix.

Smear test A few flaky cells are scraped painlessly off the surface of the cervix and examined under a microscope for abnormal shapes.

Speculum A duck-billed instrument for opening up the vagina and viewing the cervix.

Squamous cells Cells which cover the surface of the cervix. They are formed into a tough sheet of many layers of cells, resembling skin.

Stage The degree of spread of a cancer.

Steriods A group of naturally occurring compounds that may act as hormones, which are used for their ability to reduce inflammation.

Stroma cells The supportive tissue of an organ.

Subclinical Description of a disease that is suspected, but which is not sufficiently developed to produce definite signs and symptoms in the patient.

Synergestic effect A combination of factors working together, where the net result is greater than the sum of the effects of each of the factors used separately.

Synthesis The building up of complex substances by the union of simpler materials.

Tamoxifen An anti-oestrogen drug which can produce a remission in breast cancer in women (and men) of any age, and is also useful in uterine cancer.

Thermography A photograph of the breasts, showing areas of increased heat.

T-lymphocytes White blood cells from the thymus gland which are involved in the rejection of transplants of organs or tissue.

Transformation zone An area on the surface of the cervix in which the original squamous cells are replaced by columnar cells.

Trimester Three month period.

Tylectomy Another term for lumpectomy, the removal of the affected part of a cancerous breast and a few armpit lymph nodes for testing.

Ultrasound scan A technique where sound waves produce a picture of the abdominal area.

Uterine adnexia Those parts which adjoin the uterus: the ovaries and Fallopian tubes.

Uterus The pear-shaped organ, also known as the womb, in which a baby develops from a fertilised egg.

Vagina The muscular canal extending from the uterus to the outside of the body.

Vault smear Smear test taken on a woman who has had her cervix and uterus removed and the far end of her vagina sewn up. The smear is taken at the far end of the vagina because if the cancer were to reappear, it would show up here first.

Vulva The two pairs of fleshy folds (the labia majora and labia minora) that surround the openings of the vagina and urethra and extend forward to the clitoris.

Wart virus or human papilloma virus (HPV) A general term for a whole group of viruses which cause warts in different parts of the body. Only two to three kinds of genital warts are thought to be associated with cervical cancer.

Xerography A special X-ray that outlines the structures of the breast.

X-ray High-energy radiation used in high doses to treat cancer, or in low doses to diagnose the disease. Abnormal growths show up darker than normal organs.

Useful Addresses

THE MAIN ORTHODOX AND COMPLEMENTARY CANCER HELP ORGANISATIONS

England

Association of New Approaches to Cancer (ANAC), c/o Park Attwood Clinic, Trimpley, Bewdley, Worcs. DY12 1RE (tel: 029 97375). The first of the national cancer advisory organisations. Acts as the 'umbrella' for a national network of self-help groups and holistic practitioners. Takes a holistic approach while co-operating with orthodox doctors. Puts people in touch with their local holistic self-help group, and helps to establish such groups. Sells video tapes and books on the holistic approach; the tapes also cover relaxation, meditation and visualisation. Also gives out preventative information about cancer.

Breast Care and Mastectomy Association (BCMA), 26A Harrison Street, London WC1H 8JG (tel: 071 837 0908); In Scotland, 9 Castle Terrace, Edinburgh EH1 2DP (tel: 031 228 6715). Women volunteers who have experienced breast surgery provide information and practical advice to women who have discovered a breast lump or who have had breast surgery. Also helps with emotional problems associated with breast cancer. Offers advice on prostheses, swimwear and suitable bras, and will recommend women to other relevant organisations if need be. It is also possible to speak to volunteers who have experienced some form of complementary medicine.

British Association of Cancer United Patients and their Families and Friends (BACUP), 121-123 Charterhouse Street, London EC1M 6AA (tel: 071 608 1661; Outside London, try Freephone 0800 181199; for both numbers ring Mon to Thurs, 10am – 7pm, Friday 10am – 5.30pm). A national organisation offering information, practical advice and emotional support to cancer patients mainly on the orthodox treatments, although can refer you to complementary therapists in your area. Trained cancer nurses man the telephones, giving help and advice on all aspects of cancer treatment to patients and their family and friends. Offers an excellent series of leaflets on each of the female cancers, as well as on chemotherapy, radiotherapy, diet and the cancer patient and hair care, all free on request.

CancerLink, 17 Britannia Street, London WC1X 9JN (tel: 071 964 0260); in Scotland tel. 031 228 5557. A national information and support service mainly for cancer patients treated by orthodox methods, although will refer enquiries about complementary treatments to the relevant organisations. Helps support groups to get started, and has a directory of all such groups. Also offers emotional help. The trained staff who man the information hotline have personal or professional experience of cancer, and can deal with any aspect of the disease.

Cancer Relief Macmillan Fund, 15/19 Britten Street, London SW3 3TZ (tel: 071 351 7811). In Scotland tel: 031 229 3276. An organisation that provides help to cancer patients at all stages of the disease. Can give financial help to those cancer patients in need; an application is made on the patient's behalf by the local authority or hospital/hospice social worker. Also trains doctors and nurses, such as the Macmillan nurses, in cancer care, pain control, and emotional counselling for cancer patients and their relatives and funds the works of these nurses in the hospitals or in the community. Builds specialist 'Macmillan Units' (fourteen at present), which provide in-patient wards, home-care and day-care services for people with advanced cancer.

The Centre for Complementary Health Studies, University of Exeter, Exeter, Devon EX4 4PU (0392 433828). A new facility for the study of complementary medicine, which may soon be a major source of information on the subject. Runs two post-graduate degree courses in complementary health studies aimed at those already in the caring profession, and can provide a list of therapists UK-wide who practise the major complementary therapies (acupuncture, herbalism, homoeopathy, etc).

Council for Complementary and Alternative Medicine (CCAM), Suite 1, 19a Cavendish Square, London W1M 9AD (tel: 071 409 1440) – this organisation is concerned with the professional standards of complementary therapists. There is an information service at the same address, giving legal, educational and general information on complementary medicine.

Institute for Complementary Medicine (ICM), 21 Portland Place, London W1N 3AF (tel: 071 636 9543). Gives advice and information on all the complementary treatments. Can give you the name and address of your local homoeopath, herbalist, acupuncturist, etc. Also produces a directory of many of the professionally registered UK complementary practitioners, and has contact with other support groups. (Send an SAE.)

Women's National Cancer Control Campaign (WNCCC), 1 South Audley Street, London W1Y 5DQ (tel: 071 499 7532/4). This health education charity and national organisation is more involved with prevention, and has lists of well woman clinics all over the country where cervical smears are taken and breasts examined. Deals mostly with breast and

cervical cancers, but will refer women on when necessary. Also organises mobile screening clinics throughout Britain, which generally visit work-places. For the helplines for emotional support/information on all aspects of screening, phone 071 495 4995, Mon – Fri, 9.30am – 4.30pm.

Scotland

Tak Tent (Cancer Support Organisation), G. Block, Western Infirmary, Glasgow, Scotland, G11 6NT (tel: 041 332 3639). Provides written material and training courses for people setting up their own support groups in Scotland. Gives emotional support, counselling and information on cancers and treatments. There is a one-to-one counselling service available at the centre by appointment, and courses on 'Coping with Cancer'.

Wales

Tenovus Cancer Campaign Information Centre, 142 Whitchurch Road, Cardiff, South Wales CF4 3NA (tel: 0222 621433/619846). Provides information on all aspects of cancer, with a referral service to the appropriate cancer organisation for further help. Contact by telephone, letter or personal visit.

Northern Ireland

The Ulster Cancer Foundation, 40 – 42 Eglantine Avenue, Belfast, BT9 6DX (tel: 0232 663281/2/3; Helpline 0232 66439, 9.30am – 12.30pm, weekdays). Provides counselling and information on all aspects of cancer over the telephone, from prevention to cancer support. Operates an information helpline for cancer-related queries for patients and their families, staffed by experienced cancer nurses. Counselling at the centre can be arranged. Mastectomy advice involves volunteer visiting by former patients.

Republic of Ireland

Irish Cancer Society, 5 Northumberland Road, Dublin 4 (tel: 0001 681855 or dial '10' and ask for 'Freephone Cancer', Republic of Ireland only). Information on all aspects of cancer from nurses via Freephone service. Funds home care and rehabilitation programmes run by voluntary groups, for all cancer patients. Runs support groups for mastectomy and colostomy patients, among others. Home night nursing service available on request of patient's doctor or public health nurse.

A SELECTION OF OVARIAN CANCER SCREENING PROGRAMMES

Dr Ann Prys Davies Ovarian Cancer Screening Programme, London Hospital, Whitechapel, London E1 1BB.

Dr Peter Mason (RCOG), 27 Sussex Place, Regents Park, London N1 4RG (tel: 071 262 5425)

Dr Tom Bourne, The Ovarian Screening Clinic, King's College Hospital, Denmark Hill, London SE5 8RX (tel: 071 737 2546).

A SELECTION OF CANCER HELP CENTRES IN GREAT BRITAIN

Bournemouth Centre For Complementary Medicine (BCCM), 26 Sea Road, Boscombe, Bournemouth, Dorset BH5 1DF (tel: 0202 36354). A residential centre run by Dr Milo Siewert and Sheila Leo Siewert for both short-stay and long-term patients, using a range of complementary therapies to treat patients holistically; and cancer is only one of the conditions treated there. Diets are individually prescribed, with a strong emphasis on fresh wholefoods and vegetarian foods, vitamin, mineral and enzyme supplementation, correct breathing exercises, relaxation, detoxification treatments that include colonic irrigation enemas and special baths, and the use of some immuno-stimulants. Other natural therapies such as acupuncture, homoeopathy and spiritual healing, meditation, and cancer counselling are also on offer. Visiting therapists give talks and treatments (if desired) to the patients.

Bristol Cancer Help Centre (BCHC), Grove House, Cornwallis Grove, Clifton, Bristol BS8 4PG (tel: 0272 743216). The cancer help centre, opened in 1983, which became a role model for all the others. A dietary approach with vitamin and mineral supplementation, plus emphasis on the emotional side of cancer through therapies like counselling, meditation, visualisation, relaxation, art therapy and spiritual healing. You can visit for a day to get a taste of what it is like, or stay for five days, and you are encouraged to bring a companion to share the experience with you (check prices for this).

You can pay on BUPA, but for those in financial need, there is a bursary scheme. The DHSS will pay up to £170 of the cost when a patient is on income support. There may be short waiting lists for both day and week visits, as the centre has only nine bedrooms, four of them doubles. The diet must be strictly adhered to for three months, then the patient graduates to a less strict maintenance diet. You can watch the food being prepared and cooked in the kitchen. The centre is educational rather than medical, and is not equipped to cope with very sick patients. There are books and tapes available, and an 'introductory pack' which explains the philosophy of the centre. Patients can refer themselves, and every Monday and Friday morning there is a 'phone-in' to the resident doctors. Two-thirds of Bristol's visting patients are women, many with breast cancer. The centre is presently compiling a list of contact points.

Burrswood, Groombridge, Tunbridge Wells, Kent TN3 9PY (tel: 0892 863637). A medical healing centre set in beautiful grounds, which centres itself on the Catholic faith. Care is provided for a wide range of medical and post-operative conditions, although you will need a letter from your GP or specialist. A bursary fund is available for those in financial need.

Marie Curie Cancer Care, 28 Belgrave Square, London SW1 8QG (tel: 01 235 3325 ask for information officer). There are eleven Marie Curie Homes for long- or short-stay care for cancer patients throughout the UK – admission to a home is through the matron in charge. There is also a community nursing service (4,000 Marie Curie nurses care for cancer patients in their own homes); a nurse can be obtained through NHS Community Nursing Offices, or via the above address.

Morecambe Bay Cancer Help Centre, 11 College Road, Windermere, Cumbria LA23 1BU (tel: 09662 2548). Founded by breast cancer patient Bea Vernon in 1983 along the lines of the Bristol Centre, which Bea was involved in. No attempt is made to replace chemotherapy or radiotherapy, but the aim is to strengthen a patient's inner resources to fight disease. Once a month up to seventy patients and their relatives or friends share a day of meditation, relaxation, dance therapy and gourmet food. 'Quality of life' is the theme. Patients are encouraged to put together their own package of treatments similar to what is being offered at the BCHC.

Park Attwood Therapeutic Centre, Trimpley, Bewdley, Worcs DY12 1RE (tel: 029 97444). Opened in 1979, this registered nursing and residential home accommodates nineteen patients, staffed by qualified doctors, nurses and therapists who follow Rudolph Steiner's anthroposophical approach. It offers anthroposophical medicine such as Iscador, as well as homoeopathic, herbal and orthodox remedies. The diet is basically lacto-vegetarian, and the treatments on offer include special rhythmical massage aimed at harmonising the breathing, circulation and digestion, pyrogenic (warmth-creating) baths using plant oils, movement/speech therapy in the form of Eurthmy, and art therapy. A letter from your GP is required for a stay ranging from three days to three months. Patients pay according to their ability. Anthroposophical doctors are medically qualified first and then take additional training from the School of Spiritual Science in Switzerland.

Springhill Cancer Centre and Hospice, Cuddington Road, Dinton, Nr Aylesbury, Bucks HP18 0AD (tel: 0296 748432/748278). A converted eighteenth-century farmhouse, offering inpatient and outpatient care, which provides a place to rest between periods of active treatment. It sees itself as an extension of orthodox therapies, but offers the following therapies: counselling, visualisation, massage, physiotherapy, hydrotherapy, aromatherapy, psychotherapy and spiritual healing. Also on offer are muscle relaxation and pain control; horticultural therapy, spinning, knitting, weaving, woodwork and art. The principal, Dr Nadia Coates, has been influenced by the work of Rudolph Steiner. No charges are made.

Wellspring Clinic Ltd, 1 Coniger Road, Parsons Green, London SW6 3TB (tel: 071 736 3367). Not a residential centre but a clinic treating outpatients, run by therapist Lola de Gelabert. Cancer is only one of the ailments treated here. First, an assessment is given of the patient based on her nutritional, medical and psychological history, to determine what treatment is required. On offer are dietary advice, vitamin and mineral supplementation, colonic therapy, counselling, radionic hair analysis to determine food allergies and intolerances, energy medicine, magnetic field therapy, homoeopathy, herbal tonics acupuncture, chiropractic, reflexology, Oriental massage (Shiatsu), aromatherapy, polarity therapy, skin treatments, etc. All of these therapies can augment orthodox treatments. A referral system is used should other therapies be deemed expedient.

FURTHER ORGANISATIONS, CENTRES AND CONTACTS

Listing is by subject. Bodies not fitting into a particular group are listed alphabetically by name. E.g. the Contreras Clinic follows the section on Colonics.
NB: There are more than 300 registered self-help groups in Britain.

Acupuncture

British Medical Acupuncture Society, Newton House, Newton Lane, Warrington, Cheshire (tel: 092 573 720). For medically qualified doctors trained in acupuncture. Will send a list of members, but you need to be referred by your GP.

Council for Acupuncture, Suite 1, 19a Cavendish Square, London W1M 9AD (tel: 071 409 1440). Send £1 and an SAE for a list of lay practitioners. Member organisations include **British Acupuncture Association & Register, International Register of Oriental Medicine, Register of Traditional Chinese Medicine** and **Traditional Acupuncture Society.**

Register of Chinese Herbal Medicine, 98b Hazelville Road, London N19 (tel: 071 281 5869). Headed by acupuncturist David Lurie, this organisation will put you in touch with acupuncturists who also use Chinese herbs.

Association of Carers, 1st Floor, 21 – 23 New Road, Chatham, Kent ME4 4QJ. A national organisation offering support to relatives in the way of practical advice and contacts for local self-help groups.

Auchenkyle Health Centre, South Wood Road, Troon, Ayreshire, Scotland (tel: 0292 311414).

Bio-feedback

Audio Ltd, 26 – 28 Wendell Road, London W12 9RT (tel: 01 743 1518/4352). Rents various bio-feedback machines (mailed anywhere) on a daily or monthly basis, and gives training from the office. Also for rent is the therapeutic strobe, which gives off pulsed light and can be used in conjunction with bio-feedback machines to promote relaxation, develop imagery and encourage a sense of improved well-being.

Breathing exercises

Information on breathing exercises can be obtained from the Bristol Cancer Help Centre; there are also some listed in Penny Brohn's book, *The Bristol Programme,* and Shirley Harrison's book, *New Approaches To Cancer.*

Brighton Cancer Prevention Foundation, 6 New Road, Brighton, Sussex B1N 1UF (tel:

0273 727213). Founded by Dr Jan de Winter, this is a walk-in clinic for advice on cancer prevention. Dr de Winter stresses the importance of good nutrition, peace of mind and exercise.

British Colostomy Association, 38 – 39 Eccleston Square, London SW1V 1PB (tel: 01 828 5175). An information, advisory and emotional support service, from those with long experience of living with a colostomy. Free leaflets, list of local contacts, visits to home or hospital on request.

British Holistic Medical Association, 179 Gloucester Place, London NW1 6DX (tel: 071 262 5299). Formed in 1983 for doctors and healthcare workers. Associate membership open to the public for a £10 annual subscription. The organisation seeks to encourage orthodox doctors to use alternative therapies as an adjunct to orthodox treatment. It has a number of local groups throughout the country where you can find out more about complementary therapies; also, doctors will give advice through the post or by telephone one day a week.

Bromelain

Available from **Nutritec,** 17 Pershire Road South, Kings Norton, Birmingham B30 3EE.

BUPA, Provident House, Essex Street, London WC2R 3AX (tel: 071 353 5212). Ask for leaflets in 'The Facts About . . .' series, including *The Facts About Cancer* and *The Facts About Breasts.*

Burton, Dr Laurence, Immunology Research Center, Box F2689, Freeport, Grand Bahama Island, Bahamas (tel: 809 352 7455).

Burzynski, Dr Stanislaw, 6221 Corporate Drive, Houston, Texas 77036, USA (tel: 713 526 5662).

Cancer Aftercare and Rehabilitation Society (CARE), 21 Zetland Road, Redland, Bristol BS6 7AH (tel: 0272 427419). An organisation of cancer patients and their relatives and friends, offering advice and support. It has a 'phone-link' service and forty-seven branches throughout the country. Offers social outlets as well as informative activities.

Cancer Aid and Listening Line, Gaddum Centre, 274 Deansgate, Manchester (tel: 061 434 9163/8668).

Cancercare Lancaster, Lancaster Royal Infirmary, Ashton Road, Lancaster LA1 4RP (tel: 0524 381820).

Cancer Prevention Society, 25 Wellington Street, Glasgow, Scotland.

Carers' National Association, 29 Chilworth Mews, London W2 3RG (tel: 071 724 7776).

Offers information and advice, including contacts for local groups. Links carers with each other and encourages self-help. Also lobbies the government on behalf of carers.

Centre for the Study of Alternative Therapies, Bedford Place, Southampton, SO1 2DG.

Colonics

Colonics International Association, c/o Dr Milo Siewert, Chairman, 26 Sea Road, Boscombe, Bournemouth, Dorset BH5 1DF (tel: 0202 36354).

International Colonic Hydrotherapy Foundation, Moira Shiffron, Chairwoman, 11 Southampton Road, London NW5 4JS (tel: 071 485 7122).

Contreras Clinic (Dr Ernestos Contreras), Clinico del Mar, Tijuana, Mexico.

Counselling

British Association of Psychotherapists, 121 Hendon Lane, London N3 3PR (tel: 071 346 1747). Practitioners mostly in London and the home counties.

British Association for Counselling, 37a Sheep Street, Rugby, Warwicks CV21 3BX (tel: 0788 78328/9). Publishes a national directory which lists counsellors, psychotherapists and sources of help for psychosexual problems, free of charge. Send an SAE.

Chelsea Pastoral Foundation, 155a Kings Road, London SW3 (tel: 071 351 0839). Has a special cancer counselling project.

CRUSE (Bereavement Care), Cruse House, 126 Sheen Road, Richmond, Surrey TW9 1UR (tel: 01 940 4818). Helps any bereaved person by providing counselling individually and in groups by trained counsellors. Advice and information on practical problems, and social contact. Publications list available.

Institute of Family Therapy, 43 New Cavendish Street, London W1M 7RG (tel: 01 935 1651). Offers free counselling to recently bereaved families, or those with seriously ill family members (through its Elizabeth Raven Memorial Fund), working with the whole family. The service is free, but voluntary donations are welcomed to help other families.

MIND, The Association For Mental Health, 22 Harley Street, London W1N 2ED. Produces a psychotherapy list; send a large SAE marked 'Psychotherapy list', to the association's Information Unit.

Psychosexual Unit, Royal Maudsley Hospital, Denmark Hill, London SE5 8A2 (tel: 071 703 6333). Part of the NHS.

RELATE (formerly The National Marriage Guidance Council), Herbert Gray College, Little Church Street, Rugby CV21 3AP (tel: 0788 73241). Will give you the telephone number and address of your nearest local branch. Individual or family counselling is on offer, as well as sexual counselling for one or both partners. Payment is on a sliding scale.

Tavistock Centre, 120 Belsize Lane, London N3 (tel: 071 435 7111). Medical psychotherapy on offer for the patient and her family; referral needed by GP or consultant. Part of the NHS.

Westminster Pastoral Foundation, 23 Kensington Square, London W8 5HN (tel: 071 937 6956). An organisation that originated from the Church of England, but not a religious organisation. Offers counselling; has affiliated centres in other parts of the country. Self-referral; payment according to means.

The Women's Therapy Centre, 6 Manor Gardens, London N7 (tel: 071 263 6200). Offers female counselling with a political understanding of the woman's conventional role in society. Send an SAE for list of counsellors.

CYANA, 31 Church Road, London E12 6AD (tel: 081 533 5366). An East London cancer support group, run *by* cancer patients *for* cancer patients. Supplies information on treatment options in the form of leaflets and cassettes, and books from its library. Views complementary therapies as a useful back-up to orthodox treatments. Offers a twenty-four hour phone service and a once-a-week 'drop in' day.

Ecoropa UK Ltd, Ecology Action Group for Europe, Henbant Fach, Llanbedr, Crickhowell, Powys, Wales (tel: 0873 810758). Information on cancer prevention, nutrition, additives and diet.

Enzymes.

For enzyme preparations, contact **Nutritec,** 17 Pershore Road South, Kings Norton, Birmingham B30 3EE. The company's Nutrizyme tablets are made from 100 per cent selectively bred wheat sprouts, which contain enzymes that devour free radicals.

FACT (Food Additives Campaign Team), Room W, 25 Horsell Road, London N5 1XL.

Friends of Shanti Nilaya, PO Box 212, London NW8 7NW; or Old Cherry Orchard, Forest Row, East Sussex (Tel: 041 226 4626). This organisation, based on the work of Dr Elizabeth Kubler-Ross, holds workshops for the dying and the bereaved, to help them come to terms with their grief.

Gerson Diet. Information from one of the following:
(a) c/o Ms Margaret Strause (Gerson's grand-daughter), 87 Via Nazionale, 22050 – Colico (Coma) Italy.
(b) c/o Charlotte Gerson (Gerson's daughter), Gerson Institute, PO Box 430, Bonita, California 92002, USA (tel: 619 267 1150).
(c) ANAC, c/o Park Attwood, Trimpley, Bewdley, Worcs DY12 1RE (tel: 029 97375).

Gold, Dr Joseph, Syracuse Cancer Research Institute, 600 E. Genese Street, Syracuse, New York 13202, USA.

Health Education Authority, Hamilton House, Mabledon, London WCH 9TX. (tel: 071 631 0930). Provides public health information, including information about breast cancer and the National Breast Screening Programme. Ask for the leaflet *A Guide to Examining Your Breasts.*

Help For Health, South Block, Southampton General Hospital, Southampton SO9 4XY (tel: 0703 777222, ext. 3753; or 0703 779091).

Henry Doubleday Research Association, National Centre For Organic Gardening, Ryton-on-Dunsmore, Coventry CV8 3LG (tel: 0203 303517).

Herbalism
British Herbal Medicine Association, PO Box 304,

Bournemouth, Dorset BH7 6JZ (tel: 0202 433691). For lay people to join.

General Council and Register of Consultant Herbalists, Marlborough House, Swanpool, Falmouth, Cornwall TR11 4HW (tel: 0326 317321). For an SAE, will provide a short list of registered medical herbalists (with MRH after their name) in your area.

National Institute of Medical Herbalists, PO Box 3, 41 Hatherley Road, Winchester, Hants SO22 6RR (tel: 0962 68776). Enclose a large SAE for a free directory of qualified practitioners. Members have 'MNIMH' or 'FNIMH' after their names.

Homoeopathy

British Homoeopathic Association, 27a Devonshire Street, London W1N 1RJ (tel: 071 935 2163). For an SAE, the association will send you a list of medical doctors with homoeopathic training. Members have 'MFHom' after their name. They are associated with the Royal London Homoeopathic Hospital.

Hahnemann Homoeopathic Society, Humane Education Centre, Avenue Lodge, Bounds Green Road, London N22 4EU (tel: 081 889 1595). Promotes homoeopathy in Britain in general, and provides information on

it. Also publishes a magazine, *Homoeopathy Today.*

Society of Homoeopaths, 2 Artizan Road, Northampton NN1 4HU (tel: 0604 21400). Has a list of qualified lay homoeopaths – that is, homoeopaths who are not doctors, but who take a four-year course.

Royal London Homoeopathic Hospital, Great Ormond Street, London WC1 3HC (tel: 071 837 3091). There is one doctor treating cancer there, using homoeopathy as an adjunct to orthodox treatments. You will need a letter from your GP.

Hospice Information Service, St Christopher's Hospice, 51 – 59 Lawrie Park Road, London SE26 6DZ (tel: 081 778 1240/9252). Provides information about hospice-style care available in Britain and the Republic of Ireland. A full directory is available if a large SAE is sent.

Hysterectomy Support c/o The Women's Health and Reproductive Rights Information Centre, 52 Featherstone Street, London EC1Y 8RT (tel: 041 251 6332/6580, 11am – 5pm, Mon, Wed – Fri). Provides information before the operation, and can put you in touch with your local hysterectomy support group. Women (and their partners and family) are referred to former patients in their area, who will provide advice, encouragement and support through the informal sharing of experience and information – contact through letter, by telephone, or by group meetings. Booklet available.

Imperial Cancer Research Fund, PO Box 123, 44 Lincoln's Inn Fields, London WC2 3PX (tel: 071 242 0200). In the forefront of investigating every aspect of health and environment which could have a bearing on cancer.

Laetrile

Write to **Leon Chaitow,** either c/o Thorsons Publishers, Denington Estate, Wellingborough, Northants; or c/o PO Box 41, Corfu, Greece, where Leon Chaitow presently resides.

Livingston-Wheeler, Dr Virginia, Livingston Medical Centre, 3232 Duke Street, San Diego, California 92110, USA (tel: 619 224 3515).

Macmillan Nurses, c/o National Society for Cancer Relief, Anchor House, 15 – 19 Britten Street, London SW3 3TY (tel: 071 351 7811).

Macrobiotics, Community Health Foundation, 188 Old Street, London EC1V 9BP (tel: 071 251 4076).

Marie Curie Memorial Foundation, 28 Belgrave Square, London SW1X 8QG (tel: 071 235 3325). A national charity running eleven residential homes providing care for the dying; also offers nursing services for the dying in local communities, free of charge.

Meditation

School of Meditation, 158 Holland Park Avenue, London W11 4UH.

Siddha Meditation Centre, SYDUK, Campenton, Riverside Temple Gardens, Staines, Middx. TW18 3NS (tel: 0784 8164962).

Your local **Education Authority** will also provide information about meditation courses it holds in your area.

National Consumer Council, Grosvenor Gardens, London SW1.

Natural Health Clinic, 133 Gatley Road, Gatley, Cheadle, Cheshire (tel: 061 428 4980). Opened in 1969, this must be the oldest clinic offering alternative cancer therapies. It is run by Norman Eddie, a naturopath/osteopath, and offers an approach to diet which includes some of Gerson's and some of Kelley's ideas, the use of pancreatic enzymes, laetrile, Iscador, coffee enemas, herbal baths, the Hoxsey herbal treatments, electromagnetic therapy, visualisation, counselling, meditation and more.

Natural Medicines Society, Edith Lewis House, Back Lane, Ilkestone, Derby, DE7 8ET.

Natural Pure Water Association, Bank Farm, Aston Pigott, Westbury, Shrewsbury SY5 9HH (tel: 074 383 445).

Naturopathy

British Naturopathic and Osteopathic Association, 6 Netherhall Gardens, London NW3 5RR (tel: 071 435 7830). For £1 and an SAE will send a list of practitioners.

Organic Growers Association, Aeron Park, Llangeitho, Dyfed, Wales (tel: 0272 299800).

Relaxation

London Autogenic Training Centre, 101 Harley Street, London W1N 1DF (tel: 01 935 1811). Autogenic training involves a series of mental exercises to help switch off the body's 'fight or flight' reflex and to help switch on rest and relaxation. It can deal with depression, tension and hostility, among other problems.

Relaxation For Living, Dunesk, 29 Burwood Park Road, Walton-on-Thames, Surrey KT12 5LH (tel: 0932 227826).

Lifeskills, 3 Brighton Road, London N2 8JU (tel: 081 346

9646). For relaxation tapes and books.

The Bristol Cancer Help Centre and the ANAC also have relaxation tapes and books.

Research Council for Complementary Medicine, Suite 1, 19a Cavendish Square, London W1M 9AD (tel: 071 493 6930). Primarily a research organisation, but will answer your queries and refer you on to the relevant alternative organisation.

Royal Marsden Hospital Patient Education Group, Royal Marsden Hospital, Fulham Road, London SW3 6JJ (tel: 071 352 8171, ext. 437). Ask about the 'Patient Information' series of leaflets.

Rudolph Steiner House (Anthroposophical Medical Association), 35 Park Road, London NW1 6XT (tel: 071 723 4400).

Soil Association, 86 Colston Street, Bristol BS1 5BB (tel: 0272 290661).

Spiritual healing

Centre For Health and Healing, St James's Church, Piccadilly, London W1.

Matthew Manning Centre, 39 Abbeygate Street, Bury St Edmunds, Suffolk IP33 1LW (tel: 0284 69502/2364).

National Federation of Spiritual Healing, Old Manor

Farm Studio, Church Street, Sunbury-on-Thames, Middx. TW16 6RG(tel: 09327 83164). Make enquiries to the Secretary.

Spiritualist Association of Great Britain, 33 Belgrave Square, London SW1.

Sue Ryder Foundation, Sue Ryder Home, Cavendish, Suffolk CO10 8AY (tel: 09787 280252). A national charity which runs a number of homes, including several for those with advanced cancer.

Vegan Society, 33 – 35 George Street, Oxford OX1 2AY. (tel:0865 5722166).

Vegetarian Society, Parkdale, Dunham Road, Altrincham WA14 4QG (tel: 061 928 0793).

Well Woman Clinic, Family Planning Association (now a private organisation), 27 – 35 Mortimer Street, London W1N 7RJ (tel: 071 636 7866).

Wessex Cancer Help Centre, 8 South Street, Chichester, West Sussex PO19 1EH (tel: 0243 778516). Modelled on the Bristol Centre, it opened in the same year (1983). There is a growing team of practitioners – orthodox doctors, psychotherapists, homoeopaths, acupuncturists – who work with a volunteer staff there. Emphasis is on diet. Also has a list of what are believed to be

'cancer triggers', and substitutes for them. Healthy people can seek preventative advice from the centre.

World Federation for Cancer Care, 28 Belgrave Square, London SW1X 8QG (tel: 071 235 3325). Information on all cancer contacts worldwide.

Women's Health and Reproductive Rights, Information Centre, 52 Featherstone Street, London EC1 (tel: 071 251 6332). Provides information and leaflets about all aspects of women's health (including abnormal smears and cervical cancer, genital warts, breast cancers, etc.) in English and some Asian languages. Provides contact with other women who had have abnormal smears. Has a large library of books and articles, and lists of support groups and other health groups.

Women's Health Concern, Ground Floor, 17 Earl's Terrace, London W8 6LP (tel: 071 602 6669). A counselling service on all gynaecological problems; all letters with an SAE enclosed are answered.

Women's Natural Health Centre, 1 Hillside, Highgate Road, London NW5 1QT (tel: 071 482 3293). For women on a low income only and their children. Offers treatment from a herbalist, acupuncturist, osteopath, two psychotherapists; therapies include reflexology, massage, visualisation and spiritual healing as well. Payment scaled for low incomes. Ring for appointments only, 9.30am – 1.00pm.

CANADIAN CANCER SOCIETY – NATIONAL AND DIVISIONAL OFFICES

National Office, Mr Doug Barr, Chief Executive Officer, 77 Bloor Street West, Suite 1702,Toronto M5S 3A1 (tel: 416 961 7223).

Alberta & NWT Division, Mrs Margaret Partridge, Executive Director, 2424 4th Street S.W., 2nd Floor, Calgary T2S 2T4 (tel: 403 228 4487).

Manitoba Division, Mr Murray Bater, Executive Director, 193 Sherbrook Street, Winnipeg R3C 2B7 (tel: 204 774 7483).

Newfoundland & Labrador Division, Mr Harry Lake, Executive Director, P.O. Box 8921, Chimo Building, 1st Floor, Freshwater & Crosbie Road, St. John's A1B 3R9 (tel: 709 753 6520).

Ontario Division, Ms. Dorothy Lamont, Executive Director, 1639 Yonge Street, Toronto M4T 2W6 (tel: 416 488 5400).

Quebec Division, Mme. Nicole Magnan, Executive Director, Maison de la Societe, Canadienne du Cancer, Division du Quebec, 5151 Boul. L-Assomption, Montreal H1T 4A9 (tel: 514 255 5151).

Metro District, 2 Carleton Street, Suite 710, Toronto M5B 2J2 (tel: 416 593 1513).

National Public Issues Office, Mr Ken Kyle, Director, Public Issues, 77 Metcalfe Street, Suite 708, Ottawa K1P 5L6 (tel: 613 234 9539).

British Columbia & Yukon Division, Mrs Phyllis Hood, Executive Director, 565 West 10th Avenue, Vancouver, V5Z 4J4 (tel: 604 872 4400).

New Brunswick Division, Mrs Becky Boyer, Executive Director, P.O. Box 2098, 63 Union Street, Saint John E2L 3T5 (tel: 506 634 3180).

Nova Scotia Division, Mr Harley Marchand, Executive Director, 201 Roy Building, 1657 Barrington Street, Halifax B3J 2A1 (tel: 902 423 6183).

Prince Edward Island Division, Mrs Susan Loucks, Executive Director, P.O. Box 115, 131 Water Street, 2nd Floor, Charlottetown C1A 1A8 (tel: 902 566 4007).

Saskatchewan Division, Mr George Thomas, Executive Director, 2445 13th Avenue, Suite 201, Regina S4P 0W1 (tel: 306 757 4260).

ORGANISATIONS IN AUSTRALIA, NEW ZEALAND AND SOUTH AFRICA

Australia

Cancer Help

Australian Cancer Society, 155 King Street, Sydney, NSW 2000 (tel: 02 231 3355).

Cancer Information & Support Society, 14 Herberton Avenue, Hunters Hill, NSW 21110 (tel: 02 817 1912).

Sydney Square Diagnostic Breast Clinic, Breast Clinic Division, 2nd Floor, St Andrew's House, Sydney Square, Sydney NSW 2000 (tel: 02 264 7388).

Counselling

Institute of Private Clinical Psychologists of Australia, 135 Macquarie Street, Sydney NSW 2000 (tel: 02 241 1688).

New South Wales Association for Mental Health, 194 Miller Street, North Sydney, NSW 2060 (tel: 02 929 4388).

Alternative Organisations

A Course In Miracles, 47 The Point Road, Woolwich, NSW 2110 (tel: 02 817 2635).

Acupuncture Association of Australia, 5 Albion Street, Harris Park, NSW 2150 (tel: 02 633 9187).

Acupuncture Ethics and Standards Organisation, 5th Floor, 620 Harris Street, Ultimo, NSW 2007 (tel: 02 212 5250).

Association of Self-Help Organisations & Groups, 39 Darghan Street, Glebe, NSW 2037 (tel: 02 660 6136).

Australian Centre of Homoeopathy, 41 Murray Street, Tanunda, SA 5352 (tel: 085 63 2932).

Australian Institute of Homoeopathy, PO Box 122, Roseville, NSW 2069 (tel: 02 407 2876).

Australian Meditation Centre, 175 Elizabeth Street, Sydney, NSW 2000 (tel: 02 267 6274).

Australian Natural Therapists Association Ltd, 8 Thorpe Street, Woronora, NSW 2232 (tel: 02 521 2063).

Australian Vegetarian Society, 25 Ainslie Street, Kingsford, NSW 2032 (tel: 02 349 4485).

Collective of Self-Help Groups, 65 Gertrude Street, Fitzroy, Vic 3065 (tel: 03 417 6266).

Dorothy Hall College of Herbal Medicine, 558 Darling Street, Rozelle, NSW 2039 (tel: 02 818 4233).

Hopewood Health Centre Pty Ltd, Greendale Road, Wallacia, NSW 2750 (tel: 047 73 8401).

International Meditation Society, 8 Bannerman Street, Cremorne, NSW 2090 (tel: 02 909 3199).

National Herbalist Association of Australia, 2 Duffy Avenue, Kinsgrove, NSW 2208 (tel: 02 787 4523).

Swami Sarasvati Rejuvenation Centre, 185 Pitt Town Road, Kenthurst NSW 2154 (tel: 02 654 9030). For meditation.

Western Institute of Self-Help, 80 Railway Road, Cottlesloe, WA 6011 (tel: 09 393 3188).

Woman's Stress Resource Centre, 112 West Botany Road, Arncliffe, NSW 2205 (tel: 02 59 4251).

NEW ZEALAND

Cancer

Cancer Society of New Zealand, 41 Gillies Avenue, Auckland 3.

Alternative Organisations

Australasian College of Herbal Studies, Hillside Road, Ostend, Waiheke.

Epsom Counselling Services, 676 Ranfurly Road, Epsom, Auckland 3.

Homoeopathy Department, Lincoln Grove Health Centre, 292 Lincoln Road, Henderson.

New Zealand Association of Medical Herbalists, ASB Chambers, 139 Queen Street, Auckland.

New Zealand Clinic of Acupuncture, 1st Floor, APC House, 24 High Street, Auckland.

New Zealand Psychological Society, PO Box 4092, Wellington.

Peking Chinese Acupuncture Institute, 506 Queen Street, Auckland.

Psychological and Hypnotic Therapeutics, Institute of New Zealand, PO Box 2054, Auckland.

South Pacific College of Naturopaths and Therapeutics, 10 Arthur Street, Ellerslie, Auckland 6.

SOUTH AFRICA

Homoeopaths, naturopaths and herbalists are covered by the following organisation:

South African Homoeopathic Association, PO Box 10255, Strubenvale, 1570 (tel: Johannesburg 011 565121).

Bibliography

About Laetrile, Leon Chaitow (Thorsons, 1979).

Acupuncture: From Ancient Art to Modern Medicine, A. Macdonald (Unwin Paperbacks, 1984).

Alternative Healthcare for Women, Patsy Westcott (Grapevine, 1987).

The Alternative Health Guide, Brian Inglis and Ruth West (Michael Joseph, 1983).

Alternative Medicine, Dr Andrew Stanway (Penguin, 1986)

Alternatives in Healing, Simon Mills, consultant editor (Macmillan, 1988).

The Anatomy of an Illness, Norman Cousins (Bantam, 1981).

Blessed by Illness, L.F.C. Mees (Anthroposophic Press, 1983).

Breast Cancer: The Facts, Michael Baum (Oxford University Press, 1988).

Breast Cancer - A Guide to its Early Detection and Treatment, Caroline Faulder (Pan, 1979).

Breast Cancer (Your Questions Answered), Pat Webb and Marilyn Marks (Lederle Laboratories, Fareham Road, Gosport, Hants PO13 0AS).

The Bristol Diet, Alec Forbes (Century Paperbacks, 1984).

The Bristol Programme, Penny Brohn (Century Paperbacks, 1987).

British Herbal Pharmacopoeia (British Herbal Medical Association, 1983).

Cancer and its Nutritional Therapies, R.A. Passwater (Keats Publishing Inc. 1986).

Cancer and Leukaemia – An Alternative Approach, Jan De Vries (Brainstream Publishing Co., 1988).

Cancer and Vitamin C, Ewan Cameron and Linus Pauling (Warner Books Inc., 1981). Obtainable from 75 Rockefeller Plaza, New York, NY 10019, USA.

Cancer: How to Prevent It and How to Help Your Doctor Fight It, George E. Berkley, PhD (Prentice Hall Inc., 1978).

The Cancer Journals, Audre Lorde (Sheba Feminist Publishers, 1980).

Cancer – The Facts, Sir Ronald Bodley-Scott (Oxford University Press, 1981).

A Cancer Therapy - Results of 50 Cases, Max Gerson, (Totality Books, 1977). Obtainable from Margaret Strause, 97 Bedford Court Mansions, London WC1; or from PO Box 1035, Del Mar, California 92014, USA.

Can You Avoid Cancer? Peter Goodwin (BBC Publications, 1984).

Caring for the Sick at Home, T.V. Bentheim (Floris, 1987).

The Causes of Cancer. Quantitative Estimates of Avoidable Risks of Cancer in the United States Today, R. Peto and R. Doll (Oxford University Press, 1981).

Chinese Medicine, Ted J. Kaptchuk (Century Paperbacks, 1988).

The College of Health Guide to Alternative Medicine, Ruth West (The College of Health, 2 Marylebone Road, London NW1 4DX).

Crackdown on Cancer with Good Nutrition, Ruth Yale Long, PhD (Nutrition Education Ass. Inc., Texas, USA).

Does Diet Cure Cancer? Dr Maud Tresillian Fere, (Thorsons, 1971).

Dr Issels and His Revolutionary Cancer Treatment, Gordon Thomas (Peter H. Wyden, 1973. Obtainable from 750 Third Avenue, New York, NY 10013 USA).

E For Additives, Maurice Hanssen, (Thorsons, 1985).

An End to Cancer, Leon Chaitow (Thorsons, 1978).

Fit For Life, Harvey and Marilyn Diamond (Bantam Paperbacks, 1987).

Food Alive: Man Alive – Diet Handbook for Cancer and Chronic Diseases, Virginia Livingston-Wheeler, MD, and Owen Webster Wheeler, MD (1977). Obtainable from Livingston-Wheeler Medical Clinic, 3232 Duke Street, San Diego, California 92110, USA.

Foods That Fight Cancer, Patricia Hansman (Ebury New Health Guides, Ebury Press, 1987).

Gary Null's Complete Guide to Healing Your Body Naturally, Gary Null (an Omni Book, McGraw-Hill, 1988).

The Gate of Healing, Ian Pearce (Spearman, 1983).

Gentle Giants, Penny Brohn (Century Paperbacks, 1987).

A Gentle Way With Cancer, Brenda Kidman (Arrow Books, 1986).

Getting Well Again, Dr Carl and Stephanie Simonton (Bantam Books, 1986).

The Holistic Approach to Cancer, Dr Ian Pearce (ANAC, 1980).

The Holistic Herbal, David Hoffman (Element Books, 1988).

Homoeopathy. A Patient's Guide, A. Clover (Thorsons, 1984).

How to Avoid Cancer, Dr Jan de Winter (Javelin Books, 1985).

How to Live Longer and Feel Better, Dr Linus Pauling (W.H. Freeman Books, 1986).

How to Meditate, Lawrence Le Shan (Thorsons, 1983).

In Our Own Hands: Book of Self-Help Therapy, Sheila Ernst and Lucy Goodison (Women's Press, 1981).

Introduction to Homoeopathic Medicine, H. Boyd (Beaconsfield, 1981).

Living with Cancer, Jenny Bryan and Joanna Lyall (Penguin, 1987).

Living with Death and Dying, Elizabeth Kubler Ross (Souvenir, 1982).

Maximum Immunity, Michael A. Weiner, PhD (Gateway Books, 1986).

Medicine's Missing Link: Metabolic Typing and Your Personal Food Plan, Tom and Caroline Valentine (Thorsons, 1987).

The Microbiology of Cancer, Virginia Livingston-Wheeler, MD. Obtainable from Livingston-Wheeler Medical Clinic, 3232 Duke Street, San Diego, California 92110, USA.

Mind Over Cancer, Colin Ryder Richardson (Foulsham, 1988).

Naturopathic Medicine: Treating the Whole Person, Roger Newman Turner (Thorsons, 1984).

New Approaches to Cancer, Shirley Harrison (Century Paperbacks, 1987).

The Patient's Guide to Cancer Care, (Health Improvements Research Corp., New York, USA).

Risk Factors for Breast Cancer, A. Kalacho and M. Vessey (Clinics in Oncology – breast cancer, Vol. 1, no.3, p.661, ed. M. Baum, published by W.B. Saunders Co. Ltd., London, 1982).

Say No to Cancer, Barbara Waters (Nutritional Therapy, Scottsdale, New Zealand).

The Science of Homoeopathy, G. Vithoulkas (Grove Press, 1980).

A Time to Heal, Beata Bishop (Severn House, 1985).

To Live Until We Say Goodbye, Elizabeth Kubler-Ross (Prentice-Hall Inc. 1980).

Understanding Cancer (Consumer's Association, 1986).

Why Meditation, Swami Shyam (A Be All Publication, 1983).

A Woman's Guide to Alternative Medicine, Liz Grist (Fontana, 1986).

A Woman's Guide to Homoeopathic Medicine, Dr Trevor Smith (Thorsons, 1984).

You Can Fight for Your Life, Lawrence Le Shan (Thorsons, 1980).

Your Cancer, Your Life, Dr Trish Reynolds (Macdonald Optima, 1987).

INDEX